Preventive Care
Through
Home Testing

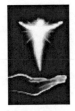

Gordin Medical Center

To my Mother,
with love and gratitude.

Preventive Care Through Home Testing

DR. VLADIMIR GORDIN

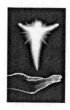

Gordin Medical Center

First published in the United States in 2012 by Gordin Medical Center
350 E. Dundee Rd., Suite 300, Wheeling, IL 60090, United States.

Every effort has been made to ensure that the information contained within this publication is accurate at the time of printing. However, this book is not an attempt by the author to render medical services to the individual reader, and should not be taken as such. This publication presents only the author's opinions, based upon his knowledge, experience and beliefs. This book is not intended to be, and must not be taken as, a replacement for consulting with your healthcare provider. Consult with a qualified healthcare provider if you are injured, or if you suffer from any medical condition. The author or publisher shall in no way be held liable or responsible for any loss or damage allegedly arising from any information contained within this book.

Author: Dr. Vladimir Gordin
Phone: (847) 243-2110
Email: info@gordinmedical.com
Websites:
www.GordinMedical.com
www.HealMeVladimir.com
www.Health1240.com

Book Design and Cover Illustration:
Writers for the Future, LLC.
Email: Writers.for.the.Future@gmail.com
Web: FutureWrit.com, AlexanderPhoenix.com

A complete listing of picture credits can be found at the back of this book.

ISBN 978-0-9856303-3-1

Dr. Vladimir Gordin

Contents

Chapter 1:

Introduction

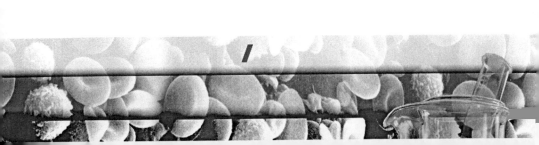

Chapter 1:

Introduction

If you opened this book, you are concerned about your health. You've most likely had to put up with traditional medicine not finding problems in time, side effects from drugs that treat only the symptoms, not the problems, and the feeling that modern medicine has failed you in one way or another.

In the following chapters, you will learn easy home tests that you can perform to monitor your health, catch problems early, and prevent them from progressing. With this book, you have taken the first step to regaining control of your health, understanding your body, and preventing disease.

Why Traditional Medicine Has Failed Us

At one time or another, you have probably gone to the doctor and wondered, "Why did this happen to me? Couldn't it have been prevented?"

The real problem in traditional medicine is that it is based on an acute care model, not a preventative care mode. This means that in traditional medicine, doctors only treat people once they are already sick rather than working to prevent disease from happening in the first place.

In modern medicine, doctors treat the symptoms, ignoring the whole person and as more symptoms come up, they treat those. It's a never ending cycle of deteriorating health for patients who are stuck in the middle.

In our world today, natural medicine and even vitamin supplements are under siege from the medical and pharmaceutical community. The goal is to convince people that living healthier, taking care of your body, and feeding your body the vitamins and nutrients it needs not only doesn't help but that it is actually dangerous.

In this way, patients will be forced to turn to traditional medicine only. And, without preventative care, more and more people will fall victim to ill health and disease daily.

How Bad Is Our Current Medical System?

The history of the medical and pharmaceutical community in our country is not a pretty one and statistics show how dangerous the reliance on traditional medicine is for patients. Doctors are supposed to be preventing and reversing disease and, as the Hippocratic Oath they take says, "First, do no harm." However, studies prove that just the opposite is in fact happening daily. There are now even many medical doctors questioning their own system and the danger it poses to patients.

In a study taking into account years of reported medical incidents, injuries, and death, a group of doctors discovered some frightening statistics.

Their study showed that in-hospital drug reactions happened at a rate of 2.2 million per year. 20 million unnecessary antibiotics are prescribed every year for viral infections. 8.9 million people per year are unnecessarily hospitalized and traditional medicine results in a staggering 783,936 deaths per year.[1]

This makes the American medical system the leading cause of death and injury in the United States, beating out heart disease and cancer.

Even worse, the group stated that their statistics were actually very low since most incidents go unreported to protect the reputation of doctors and staff.

What Went Wrong?

As anyone who has ever been to a Medical Doctor knows, you will probably be given a prescription. Whether that prescription is necessary or will help or hurt you, is another question. But,

---

[1] Null, G, PhD, Dean, C, MD, ND, Feldman, M, MD, Rasio, D, MD, Smith, D, PhD. " 2004" Death by Medicine. Retrieved May 13, 2012 from Life Extension Magazine [online copy].
www.lef.org/magazine/mag2004/mar2004_awsi_death_01.htm

there is no doubt that the pharmaceutical industry is a multi-billion dollar a year industry and is so tightly tied to the traditional medical system that the hold is unbreakable.

According to an ABC news report, pharmaceutical companies spend over $2 billion a year on over 314,000 events attended by doctors, a conflict of interest waiting to happen. The report also noted that when a pharmaceutical company funds a clinical drug trial, there is a 90% chance that the drug will pass and be released for use by the public. But, if a non-pharmaceutical company funds the trial, there is only a 50% chance that the drug will pass.[2]

So, it seems that money can buy happiness, at least for the drug companies.

Pharmaceutical companies and traditional medicine are so inseparable that they even fund medical schools and hospitals and advertise in medical journals.[3] With such a focus on the business of medicine, is it any wonder that government regulatory agencies like the FDA are touting the dangers of vitamins while ignoring the long list of side effects and dangerous statistics of prescription medications?

---

[2] McKenzie, J. "Conflict of Interest? Medical journal changes policy of finding independent contractors [transcript]. ABC News. June 12, 2002.

[3] Campbell, EG, Weissman JS, Clarridge B, Yucel, R, Causino, N, Blumenthal, D. "Characteristics of Medical School faculty members serving on institutional review boards: results of a national survey". Acad. Med. 2003. Aug; 78(8): 831-6.

Probably the biggest irony in modern medicine is that as more medicines are introduced to the market, more diseases are discovered each year. In developed countries, like the United States, more than half of people take daily prescription medication and yet our country gets more unhealthy every day.

How is Preventative Medicine Different?

While traditional medicine treats symptoms once they happen, preventative medicine works to discover underlying problems and fix them before they progress to disease. In short, traditional medicine is reactive while preventative medicine is proactive.

Preventative medicine also differs from the traditional approach in that it takes a holistic approach. It looks at the person as a whole: their bones, joints, muscles, spine, diet, nutrition, allergies, stress, anxiety, depression, fatigue, and much more. This allows for a broad based treatment and the early discovery of problems in the body so that they don't progress to dangerous diseases.

What Can You Do?

As we said previously, just by opening this book, you have taken the first step toward regaining control of your health, learning to listen to your body, and preventing disease.

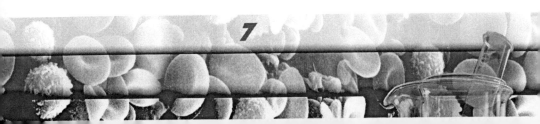

Preventive Care Through Home Testing

In this book we will take you step by step through tests, routines, and procedures that you can do at home with no medical experience to check your health status so that you can prevent disease and problems before they become serious and symptomatic.

Not only will we show you each step of the process, we will teach you why they are important, help you understand what your results mean and when you should seek professional help, and show you how to find someone that will treat the cause of your issues, not just the symptoms.

At the back of the book, you will find an easy to use workbook with charts and graphs where you can make notes and keep track of your test results and progress. Make sure to use the workbook. It is an important tool to not only help you track your health status, but is also a very important written record should you need to consult a healthcare professional for help.

Let's Get Started!

It's now time to begin your journey to a healthier, happier life. Take each chapter a step at a time, follow the instructions, and record your results.

By using this book, you will learn more about your health in a few short days than you have in all the doctors' visits you've been to in your entire life.

So, make today the first day of your new healthier life.

Chapter 2:

Your Blood Pressure and Your Health

Chapter 2:

Your Blood Pressure and Your Health

If you've ever been to the doctor, you've had your blood pressure taken. But, why is it important and how do you know when you have a problem?

Simply put, your blood pressure is the pressure your heart puts against you blood vessels as it pumps blood through your body. Your blood pressure tells you how hard your heart is working, whether or not it is able to rest between beats, and if there is a possibility of disease or blockage in your heart or blood vessels.

The Numbers

Your blood pressure is made up of two numbers. The first number (or highest number) is called the systolic. It measures how hard your heart is working when it beats. The second number, your diastolic (or lower number) measures the workload on your heart when it's at rest.

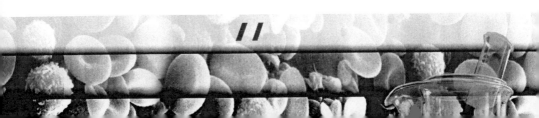

For Example: 120/80 =

120 is the systolic pressure

80 is the diastolic pressure

These two numbers together give an overall view of the health of your heart and blood vessels.

Your Blood Pressure Reading, Normal or Not?

Traditionally, normal blood pressure has been labeled as 120/80. A person has been considered to have high blood pressure if their reading is 140/90 or higher and low blood pressure at 90/60 or lower.

Blood Pressure Chart

210/120	Stage 4 High Blood Pressure
180/110	Stage 3 High Blood Pressure
160/100	Stage 2 High Blood Pressure
140/90	Stage 1 High Blood Pressure
130/85	High Normal
120/80	Normal
110/75	Low Normal
90/60	Borderline Low

Dr. Vladimir Gordin

High Blood Pressure - Causes and Symptoms

High blood presser is caused by a greater than normal pressure pushing though your arteries. There are many things that can lead to high blood pressure, most of which are preventable.

Causes of High Blood Pressure

- Smoking
- Weight Gain/Obesity
- Lack of Physical Activity
- Too Much Alcohol Consumption
- Stress
- Use of Birth Control Drugs
- Adrenal and Thyroid Disease
- Chronic Kidney Disease

Whatever the cause, high blood pressure can cause you to feel stressed, tired, bloated, and weak. And, when left untreated, can lead to stroke, heart failure, heart attack, kidney failure, vision loss, and erectile dysfunction.[4]

According to an editorial in the Lancet, the risk of high blood pressure in a developed country like the U.S. is over 90%.[5] This

---

[4] U.S. National Library of Medicine. "2012" High blood pressure. Retrieved May, 14 2012 from Medline Plus www.nlm.nih.gov/medlineplus/highbloodpressure.html
[5] Lancet 2007: 370: 539: Hypertension: uncontrolled and conquering the world. [editorial]

means that you have a 9 in 10 chance of suffering from high blood pressure at some time in your life which makes tracking and controlling your blood pressure one of the most important parts of a healthy life.

Low Blood Pressure – Causes and Symptoms

Low blood pressure can have as much of a negative effect on your health as high blood pressure so it is important to know what it's causes are and how to prevent it.

Causes of Low Blood Pressure

- Nutritional Deficiencies
- Endocrine Problems
- Irregular Heartbeat
- Medications (Including diuretics, heart medications, anti-depressants, and narcotics)
- Alcohol Consumption[6]

Low blood pressure can cause dizziness, fainting, and in severe cases can deprive your brain and body of oxygen, leading to death.

---

[6] American Heart Association. "2012" High blood pressure. Retrieved May 14, 2012 from American Heart Association www.heart.org/HEARTORG/conditions/HighBloodPressure...re_UCM_301785_Article.jsp

Dr. Vladimir Gordin

The Truth about Traditional Medicine and Blood Pressure Treatment

Your blood pressure can vary throughout the day, even hour to hour. The reading can change due to arm position, the wrong size cuff, and even because of what is known as "white coat syndrome", which is when a person's blood pressure goes up just because of the stress of being in a doctor's office. That is why it is important to monitor your blood pressure consistently over time to make sure you get an accurate baseline reading for you.

Unfortunately, in traditional medicine, even one abnormal blood pressure reading often results in a prescription being given. Patients end up on long term, often dangerous heart medications. This sets off a chain of events of more symptoms, more medications, and a higher risk of future heart problems.

Even worse, the guidelines for what are considered abnormal vs. normal blood pressure readings and when medicine should be prescribed has been heavily influenced by the drug companies themselves. Despite the many years of a 120/80 reading being considered normal, in December 2003 the JNC, the Joint National Committee on Prevention, Detection, Evaluation, and Treatment of High Blood Pressure, issued new guidelines for blood pressure readings. The guidelines stated that a systolic pressure of 120-139 is now considered pre-hypertensive (pre-high blood pressure) and suddenly created 45 million new Americans with high blood pressure who were previously considered healthy. That's a lot of new customers for the pharmaceutical companies.[7]

Sadly, a study by the British Medical Association found that 97% of people who were given drugs for high blood pressure had significant side effects.[8] And yet, in spite of the increased number of prescriptions given to treat high blood pressure, no real progress has been made in controlling it in the United States.

Even with the side effects and the lack of proven results, most people with high blood pressure are put on more than one prescription medication to treat their condition. And, Medical Doctors routinely ignore the factors of stress, lifestyle, diet, and nutrition and their effects on a patient's blood pressure readings.

---

[7] National Heart, Lung, and Blood Institute. "2003" Seventh Report of the Joint National Committee on Prevention, Detection, Evaluation, and Treatment of High Blood Pressure, Retrieved May 14, 2012 from JNC 7 Express
http://www.nhlbi.nih.gov/guidelines/hypertension/jhcintro.htm
[8] Rosch, P. "2009" Why has the treatment of hypertension become such a deplorable fiasco? Retrieved from The American Institute of Stress www.stress.org/interview-Stress_Hypertension.htm

Dr. Vladimir Gordin

How to Monitor Your Blood Pressure At Home

Now that you understand the significance of your blood pressure and the causes and symptoms that go with both high and low blood pressure, we're going to show you the proper way to monitor your own blood pressure at home.

You don't need any medical training and it only takes a few small tools to help you keep track of your blood pressure and recognize the early warning signs of disease to prevent them from becoming serious.

Tip: The one rule to remember is to always measure your blood pressure as soon as you wake up. This provides the most reliable reading, assuming that you have rested for at least 8 hours. This is very important because your blood pressure can change throughout the day based on the structural, chemical, and emotional changes in your body discussed in this chapter.

What You Need

There are two ways to take your blood pressure at home. The first and easiest is by using an automatic blood pressure cuff that fits around your wrist. The second is the use of a standard, manual blood pressure cuff and stethoscope.

Whichever you choose, they are easy to find at both pharmacies and medical supply stores.

Automatic Blood Pressure Cuff – Step by Step Use

Using an automatic blood pressure cuff is very easy. Just follow these steps.

1. Wrap the cuff around your wrist and fasten the Velcro, making sure that it feels snug but not too tight.

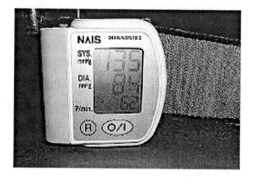

2. Keep your arm relaxed and at the level of your heart.
3. Press the "Start" button.
4. Wait while the cuff inflates and slowly deflates.
5. Check you reading.
6. Repeat on your other arm.

Tip: For the most accurate reading, avoid smoking, coffee, and heavy exercise for 30 minutes prior to taking your blood pressure. And, for five minutes prior to taking the reading, sit upright in a chair, with your legs uncrossed and your feet flat on the floor. This allows your body to return to its normal rhythm so that you get the most precise reading possible.

Manual Blood Pressure Cuff – Step By Step Use

If you decide to go with a manual blood pressure cuff, the process is a little bit more involved but if you follow these steps, you will get a very accurate reading. For this process, you need both a blood pressure cuff and a stethoscope.

1. Wrap the blood pressure cuff around your arm, right above your elbow.

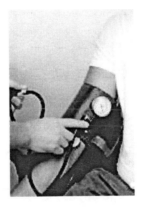

2. Put the earpieces of the stethoscope in your ears and place the bell of the stethoscope on the inside of your elbow, where your arm bends.

3. Make sure your arm is relaxed and pump the cuff to 180. Be sure that the valve is closed on the cuff by turning the silver piece clockwise until it's tight.

4. Slowly release the air while listening for the sound of a heartbeat (a thump).

5. When you hear the first thump, check the number on the gauge, this is your systolic pressure, or top number.

6. Continue listening as you let the air out until you hear the last little thump (it's very quiet). Check the number on the gauge. This is your diastolic pressure, or bottom number.

Tip: How to Choose the Right Fit for a Manual Blood Pressure Cuff

As we've talked about, the wrong size blood pressure cuff can change your reading and make it inaccurate. But, there is an easy way to make sure you pick the right size for you.

1. Sit in a chair with your elbows bent and arms resting on the armrest.

2. Using a tape measure, measure around the midpoint between your shoulder and elbow of the arm you use the least. For example, if you are right-handed, measure your left arm.

3. Record the measurement in centimeters (cm). This will tell you which size of blood pressure cuff is right for your arm.

Chart of Cuff Sizes	
Arm Circumference (cm)	Size
22-26	small adult
27-34	adult
35-44	large adult

Should You Check Both Sides?

Now that you know how to take your own blood pressure, it's important to not only check it regularly, but to check your blood pressure in both arms for differences.

Studies have shown that differences in blood pressure readings between a person's right and left arm are a reliable indicator of cardiovascular disease and even death.[9]   A small difference from side to side is normal, but a difference in readings of greater than 10mm can indicate a problem. This can often be the first sign of peripheral vascular disease, heart problems, and high blood pressure.

---

[9] Heid, M. "2012" The simple test that could save your life. Retrieved May 14, 2012 from Prevention www.prevention.com/health/health-concerns/importance-blood-pressure-testing-both-arms

What Does An Abnormal Reading Mean to You?

If after monitoring your blood pressure, you find that it is too high, too low, or that there is more than a 10 mm difference between the blood pressure in your right and left arm, you are left with the question, "What does this mean to me?"

As we've discussed, there are many things that can cause a change in blood pressure, including diet, exercise, smoking, alcohol consumption, problems with your endocrine system like your adrenal glands and thyroid, nutritional deficiencies, blockages of blood vessels, heart problems, and more.

This is why it is of the utmost importance that if your blood pressure readings are abnormal, you must seek assistance from a trained professional who will take a holistic approach to your blood pressure problems.

You don't want someone who is just going to give you a pill to treat the symptoms and never reach the cause of the problem.

A good choice is a multi-disciplinary Chiropractic practice that focuses on all aspects of the human body and their relationship to your overall health. A Chiropractic Physician is a point of entry doctor who is trained in all aspects of health and can look at your body as whole to discover the underlying cause of your blood pressure problems. Since there are so many things that can result in blood pressure changes, these professionals can analyze your diet, stress levels, nutritional problems, health history, and a host of other factors to find and treat the cause of the problem, not just the symptoms.

Treatment may include stress management, nutritional therapy, diet and exercise management, hands on chiropractic adjustments to allow the nerves to the heart to work more freely, and much more. With this holistic, proactive approach, your Chiropractic Physician can help you get control of your blood pressure and your health.

Your Homework

Now that you understand what your blood pressure means, why it is important, and how to monitor it at home, it's time to get started discovering more about your personal health level.

Your homework for this chapter is to take your blood pressure in each arm for 14 days and record the results in the workbook section at the end of the book.

If your blood pressure is normal, Congratulations! You are one step closer to a healthier life. But, don't forget to continue to check it at least once a week to make sure it remains in normal limits.

If your readings are abnormal 3 or more times in those 2 weeks or differ from side to side by more than 10mm, you now know how to find the care that is right for you. The exception to this is an extremely elevated blood pressure. In this case, seek immediate medical attention due to the risk of stroke.

What's Next?

In the next chapter, we will focus on the pulse oximetry test, how to do it, and what it means to your health.

Each step you take brings you closer to a long, healthy life. So, don't stop now.

Chapter 3:

Pulse Oximetry, Oxygen, and Your Health

Chapter 3:

Pulse Oximetry, Oxygen, and Your Health

Pulse oximetry is a simple test that can be done at home to determine whether or not your blood is carrying enough oxygen to your brain, organs, and other body tissues. Since without enough oxygen, no living organism can survive, the amount of oxygen in your blood is a very important indicator of your health.

How It Works

The color of your blood changes depending on how much oxygen it is carrying. When you use a pulse oximeter, it shines two beams of light through your finger. One light is a red light that you can see. The other is an infrared light that you won't be able to see. These lights bounce off a photodetector on the opposite side of your finger and measure the color of your blood. Based on that color, the device can determine the oxygen saturation level of your blood.

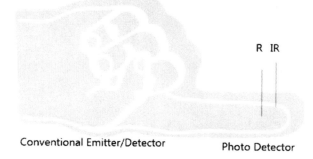

R IR

Conventional Emitter/Detector   Photo Detector

What Is Oxygen Saturation and Why Is It Important to Check?

Your oxygen is carried in your blood by hemoglobin molecules. Oxygen Saturation is a measurement of how much the hemoglobin molecules are carrying compared to how much they could carry at maximum capacity.

For example if you had 2 hemoglobin molecules that could carry a maximum of 200 oxygen molecules, or 100 each, if they were carrying 194 oxygen molecules, they would be 97% saturated. (194/200 x 100 = 97%)

The level of oxygen saturation in your body is important because it gives an initial picture of how well your lungs are working, whether or not your hemoglobin molecules are able to function at full capacity, and if your body is receiving the oxygen it needs not just to function but also to thrive. Oxygen is vital to all of your organs and tissues, including your heart and brain.

Without oxygen, hypoxia, a deprivation of oxygen, sets in and the tissues begin to die.

How to Find a Pulse Oximeter for Home Use

Today, pulse oximeters are easy to buy for use at home either from a medical supply store or through the internet. They are generally inexpensive, costing between $30 and $60 for a basic home device that will serve all your needs. A fingertip pulse oximeter is the best and easiest choice for home use for adults and will give you an accurate reading without any added difficulties. Most have only one button so you will have no difficulty figuring out how to use your pulse oximeter at home.

Using Your Pulse Oximeter – Step By Step Instructions

A fingertip pulse oximeter is very simple to use. Just follow these instructions and you will get a quick, precise reading.

1. Remove any nail polish since the lights of the pulse oximeter have a hard time passing through the polish.
2. Place the pulse oximeter on your finger. (Your index or ring finger is best.)

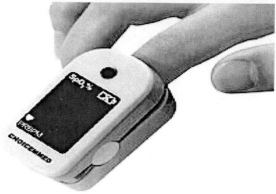

3. Rest you arm on a steady surface to prevent movement. Movement affects the reading ability of the pulse oximeter.
4. Stay still and wait for your reading. It can take a few seconds to a minute for your reading to finish.
5. Take your pulse ox reading daily to determine your normal baseline.

Tip: If you have cold hands, it can be difficult to get an accurate reading. Before using the pulse oximeter, warm your hand by wrapping it in a warm towel for a few minutes.

What Is a Normal Pulse Ox Reading?

In a normal, healthy person, their pulse oximetry reading should be between 99% and 100%. This means that their blood is 99-100% saturated with oxygen. This is especially important in children, whose oxygen level should always be close to 100%.

In adults, 98% can be acceptable if you are tired, fatigued, underfed, or otherwise compromised. Otherwise, any reading below 99% signifies that you have a slow healing ability, slow recuperation, slow regeneration, and slow detoxification.

Any reading below 99% should be given close attention and you should seek care from a qualified professional to diagnose the cause behind the low levels of oxygen in your blood and provide appropriate treatment.

What Low Readings Can Mean to You

Low levels of oxygen saturation in your blood can have many different causes, all of which need to be checked to determine the underlying issue. Living without enough oxygen for too long deprives your tissues of this needed nutrient and will cause cell damage and death.

Lung problems, heart problems, anemia affecting the hemoglobin molecules, other blood disorders, nutrient deficiencies, and improper breathing can all affect the levels of oxygen saturation in your blood. Low level of oxygen can signal the beginning of a disease process or even the presence of an already serious illness.

When and How to Seek Help

Any consistently low pulse ox readings should be further investigated to prevent a problem from becoming serious or to catch an already serious problem and target its cause.

As we talked about in the previous chapter, it is important to seek out a doctor who will take into account all aspects of your health to search for the cause of your low oxygen saturation and not just treat the symptoms. Your Chiropractic Physician can take a multi-disciplinary approach, looking at your diet, breathing, health history, exercise levels, anxiety and stress, and the health of your organs.

By taking a holistic approach they will be able to determine the cause behind the lack of oxygen in your blood and create a targeted plan to reverse the problem itself, rather than just its symptoms.

Your Homework

You now understand the importance of having a high level of oxygen to feed your body's organs and tissues. You have also learned how to use a pulse oximeter at home to monitor your oxygen saturation level to determine the status of your health and look for early warning signs of a disease process.

Your homework for this chapter is to use your pulse oximeter to take a daily reading of your oxygen saturation level and record it in the workbook at the end of the chapter. Like your blood pressure readings, you should do this daily for the next 14 days.

If your oxygen saturation levels are 99% are above, your body is receiving the oxygen it needs. But, if your readings are consistently below 99%, you now know how to find a doctor that will help you fix the cause of the problem.

What's Next?

In our next chapter, we will discuss the Allergy Pulse Diagnostic Test, what it means to your health, and how to easily perform it at home.

Every day that you make a conscious decision to work on your health adds to the quality of your life.

Chapter 4:

Allergy Pulse Diagnostic Test – How to Find Your Food Allergies at Home

Chapter 4:

Allergy Pulse Diagnostic Test – How to Find Your Food Allergies at Home

The allergy pulse diagnostic test is a simple test that is easy to perform in your own home and the only tool you need is a watch with a second hand. This test is a very useful tool to determine whether you have underlying food allergies that are negatively affecting your health and well-being.

How Food Allergies Affect Your Life

Many people suffer from allergies to food they eat every day. In fact, cow's milk is one of the most common food allergies in the United States and yet most people drink it on a daily basis. And, while most children can outgrow their food allergies, adults do not.[10]

---

[10] Stoppler, M, MD. "2012" Food allergy. Retrieved May 14, 2012 from MedicineNet.com
www.medicinenet.com/food_allergy/article.htm

Preventive Care Through Home Testing

Food allergies have been linked to many health problems that decrease the overall quality of your life. Only by eliminating these foods from your diet will your health improve.

Conditions Linked to Food Allergies[11]	
Recurrent Headache	Migraines
Nervousness	Dizziness
Constipation	Heartburn
Obesity	Irritability
Abdominal Pain	Fatigue
Indigestion	Sinusitis
Hypertension	Hives
Depression	Colitis
Conjunctivitis	Chest Pain

Many people live with these symptoms for years, never understanding why they can't find relief. But, there is no relief to be had as long as a person is still eating the foods that cause their allergic reactions.

---

[11] Coca, A, MD. " 1956" The pulse test [online copy]. Retrieved May 14, 2012 from The Soil and Health Library.
www.soilandhealth.org/02/020kyglibcat/020108.coca.pdf

Dr. Vladimir Gordin

The Difference Between Environmental and Food Allergies

For most people it is easy to recognize when they are suffering from environmental allergies. When you go outside and are exposed to specific pollen, you sneeze, your eyes water, and your nose runs. A certain time of the year, like the spring or fall always brings on the same symptoms.

With environmental allergies a skin or blood test can immediately tell you what you are or are not allergic to, from grass and cedar to cottonwood and dust mites.

With food allergies, it is not so easy. When you eat a food that you are allergic to, you may not have a reaction that is severe enough to recognize. In most cases of food allergies, you don't even know that you have them. All you know is that you feel bad. You may be tired, have headaches or indigestion, or experience any of the symptoms in the list above. The problem is that you don't know why.

And, to make matters even more difficult, traditional medicine's approach of skin and blood testing is not as effective when it comes to food allergies. With food allergies, these tests only show that you might have an allergy to a food, not whether the food is actually affecting you in a negative way. On top of that, a negative test result does not mean that you aren't allergic to that food, just that you may not have the antibody to the food at that particular time.

This makes these tests for food allergies a hit or miss prospect.

Most Common Food Allergies

There is a long list of foods to which you might have an allergy. If you are experiencing health problems, it is likely that you are eating these foods regularly and don't even know how much they are hurting your health.

Common Food Allergens

- Dairy Products
- Milk
- Sugar
- Wheat
- Gluten
- Corn
- Soy
- Nuts
- Shellfish
- Fish
- Eggs
- Peanuts
- Fruits

Dr. Vladimir Gordin

Take Control of Your Food Allergies with the Allergy Pulse Diagnostic Test

To learn what foods may be damaging your health, use the Allergy Pulse Diagnostic Test. It is an easy-to-use test that will help you single out the foods that you are allergic to so that you will be able to eliminate them from your diet and improve your overall health. When you eat a food which you are allergic to, your pulse rate increases as part of the immune response to the allergen.

According to Dr. Arthur Coca, who performed extensive testing and treatment using the Allergy Pulse Diagnostic Test, "The pulse rate in a normal person is not affected at all by digestion. It is remarkably stable. The pulse then may be considered a dependable first watchdog of our health citadel, telling us promptly whenever we are in possibly injurious contact with our allergic enemies."[12]

To perform this test, the only thing you have to know is how to take your pulse properly. You can measure your pulse rate either manually, with your fingertips, or with an automatic blood pressure cuff that also measures your pulse rate or a heart rate monitor arm band.

---

[12] Coca, A, MD. " 1956" The pulse test [online copy]. Retrieved May 14, 2012 from The Soil and Health Library. www.soilandhealth.org/02/020kyglibcat/020108.coca.pdf

Measuring Your Pulse Rate Manually

1. Place your first 2 fingers (your index and middle finger) on the palm side of your wrist at the base of your thumb.

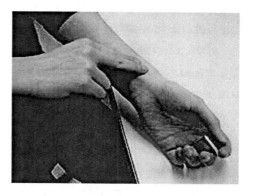

2. Gently press until you feel a beat or a pulsing. If you do not feel the pulse, adjust the placement of your fingers or switch to your other arm.
3. Using your watch, count the number of beats you feel for 60 seconds.
4. This is your pulse rate.

Tip: Some sources will tell you to take your pulse for only 10 seconds and then multiply by 6 to get your pulse rate. But, you get a much more accurate reading by counting the beats for 60 seconds as the heart rate can speed up or slow down which cannot be accounted for if you only count the beats for 10 seconds.

Choices for Monitoring Your Pulse Automatically

If you decide to measure your pulse automatically instead of with your fingertips you have two choices, both of which are easy to use, an automatic blood pressure cuff that also gives pulse readings or a heart rate monitor arm band. They are both widely available at pharmacies, medical supply stores, and over the internet.

Blood Pressure Cuff with Pulse Rate Readout

You may already have an automatic blood pressure cuff, which you have been using to chart your blood pressure readings as described in Chapter 2. Most of these cuffs will also display your pulse rate at the same time that they measure your blood pressure. With just the touch of a button, these are easy to use and a simple way to take your pulse.

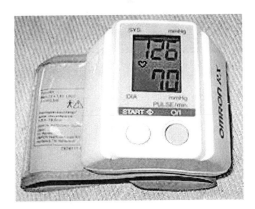

Heart Rate Monitor Armband or Wristband

Armbands with heart rate monitors are easy to use and have been used extensively to monitor a person's pulse rate during exercise. And, it's an excellent tool for keeping up with your pulse rate at home. It's easy to use and continuously monitors and calculates your heart rate.

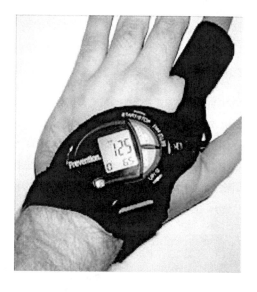

How to Perform the Allergy Diagnostic Pulse Test

1. On the day of the test, take your pulse before you get out of bed, while you are still lying down. Note the results in the Workbook.
2. Take your pulse again prior to your first meal and again record your results.
3. This meal should consist of only one type of food (one that you think you may be allergic to). You do not need to eat very much. Make sure to write down what food you ate in the workbook.
4. Take your pulse 30 minutes following the meal, recording the results, and again 60 minutes after the meal.
5. After the 60 minute pulse check, you can try a different type of food, again recording the food you ate, as well as your pulse rate after 30 and 60 minutes.
6. You can do this up to 5 times in one day. Just make sure that you record the results of your pulse rate along with the food you ate in the Workbook section provided.
7. You follow this procedure for as many days as needed to test all of the food to which you might be allergic.

Tip: Other than your morning pulse rate, which should be taken while lying down, all other readings for the day should be taken in the same position either while sitting or standing.

How to Interpret Your Results

After you have recorded all of your results and finished your testing, it is time to figure out what your results mean to you and your health. The following will help you determine if you might have a food allergy so that you will be able to seek professional help to eliminate the foods from your diet and build up your immune system.

- Any increase in pulse of more than 10 beats per minute after eating a food signals a possible food allergy.
- If your highest pulse rate is the same each day, and not over 84, you are not likely to have food allergies.
- If your maximum pulse each day varies by more than 2 beats you are probably suffering from food allergies. For example: Your highest pulse Sunday was 72, Monday 84, and Tuesday 75. There is more than a 2 beat per minute difference between these pulses.

What to Do If Your Results Indicate Food Allergies

If you have a change in your pulse rate of more than 10 beats per minute after eating a food or your maximum pulse varies more than 2 beats per minute from day to day, it is likely that you are suffering from food allergies that may be negatively impacting your health without your knowledge.

In order to restore your health, feel better, and lead a healthier life, allergen free, you will need to consult a doctor experienced in dealing with food allergies and their physical and emotional implications. Your Chiropractic Physician will be able to analyze your results and help you set up an elimination diet to confirm your food allergies. A knowledgeable Chiropractic Physician will be able to provide additional allergy testing by a variety of means. They will also be able to address other problems in your body that lead to hyperactivity of the immune system causing allergies to form.

By addressing all aspects of your health, your Chiropractic Physician will not only help you get rid of the symptoms from your food allergies but also treat the true cause to prevent your allergies from progressing in the future.

Your Homework

Understanding how food allergies can affect your health and life is the first step to beating them. Now that you know how to test for these food allergies at home, you will be able to determine what foods are most likely to cause problems for you and how to find help to overcome these allergies and get healthier.

Your homework for this chapter is to use the above guide to perform your own Allergy Pulse Diagnostic testing. Test the foods in the list of most common food allergies as well as any foods that you feel you have a negative reaction to. Make sure to record your results in your Workbook and see a qualified professional if the test reveals that you have been suffering from food allergies.

What's Next?

In the next chapter, you will learn the importance of your adrenal glands to your health and what test to use to make sure that they are functioning optimally.

All it takes to improve your health is commitment. So, decide today that you are going to live a healthier life today than yesterday.

Chapter 5:

Ragland's Test and Your Adrenal Glands

Chapter 5:

Ragland's Test and Your Adrenal Glands

You adrenal glands are extremely important to your health. They produce more than 50 hormones that help your body function properly. They are involved in energy production, fat storage, electrolyte balancing, and much more. So what happens when your adrenal glands can no longer work the way they are supposed to? And, how do you tell that you have a problem?

Fortunately, there is a simple at-home test that will let you know if you are suffering from adrenal fatigue and need to seek help. Ragland's Test is easily performed in your own home with only an automatic blood pressure cuff.

What Are Your Adrenal Glands and How Do They Work?

Your adrenal glands are part of your endocrine or hormonal system.

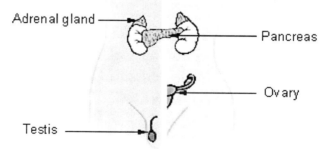

Major Endocrine Glands

Male   Female

Pituitary gland ——

—— Pineal gland

Thyroid gland ——

—— Thymus

Adrenal gland ——

—— Pancreas

—— Ovary

Testis ——

The adrenals are a very small pair of glands that sit on top of each of your kidneys. Just as you have two kidneys, you have two adrenal glands, one for each kidney. Your adrenal glands are about two inches long each while each of your kidneys are approximately the size of your fist. The adrenals are made up of two sections, the outer portion, called the cortex, and the inner portion, called the medulla.

Adrenal Gland

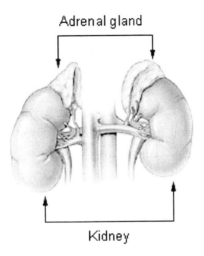

Adrenal gland

Kidney

The medulla, the inner part of your adrenal glands, makes hormones called catecholamines, like epinephrine and adrenaline. These hormones control your "fight or flight" response and affect your heart rate and sweating.

The cortex, the outer part of your adrenal glands, makes corticosteroids, androgens, and mineralocorticoids. Cortisol and aldosterone are two of the hormones made by the cortex.

These regulate the body's blood volume with the help of the kidneys, which changes your blood pressure.

The Relationship Between Your Kidneys and Your Adrenal Glands

So, as you can see, the proper functioning of your adrenal glands is very important for your health.

They produce hormones that help you deal with day-to-day stresses as well as regulate your blood pressure system and kidney function. The adrenals produce the hormones cortisol, aldosterone, norepinephrine, and many others.

Together, these hormones help to control your stress and inflammation. And, along with your kidneys, they manage your blood pressure.[13]

Renin, a chemical messenger made in your kidneys, is a signal to your adrenal glands to make three hormones: aldosterone, angiotensin I, and angiotensin II.

---

[13] Morgan, S. "2011" Adrenal glands and kidney. Retrieved May 15, 2012 from Livestrong.com www.livesrong.com/article/139350-adrenal-glands-kidneys/

Together, these hormones regulate fluid volume, the tension of the blood vessels, and the absorption of sodium. All of this has a strong, regulatory affect on your blood pressure.

The adrenal cortex (the outer portion) regulates kidney function in many ways. And, in turn, the kidneys have a regulatory effect on the adrenal glands.

Because of this feedback loop between the adrenal glands and kidneys, the health of these organs is undeniably intertwined.[14]

---

[14] Bartter, FC, Fourman P. "The different effects of aldosterone-like steroids and hydrocortisone-like steroids on urinary excretion of potassium and acid". Metabolism. 11:6, 1962 [PubMed]

What Happens When Your Adrenal Glands Aren't Working Well?

Symptoms of Adrenal Fatigue

Low Blood Sugar	Weight Gain
Low Blood Pressure	Compromised Immune System
Dizziness When Stand Up	Depression
Fatigue	Nausea and Vomiting
Foggy Thinking	Constipation
Lowered Metabolism	Abdominal Pain
Diarrhea	Changes in Skin Color
Muscle and Joint Pain	Sensitivity to Light
Loss of Scalp Hair	Excess Facial or Body Hair
Low Body Temperature	Weight Loss
Trouble Falling Asleep	Salt and Sugar Cravings
Trouble Waking Up	Need for Stimulants
Panic Attacks	Chronic Inflammation
Decreased Thyroid Function	Hot Flashes
Irritability	Mood Swings
Anxiety	Loss of Libido
Tingling in Extremities	Aching Joints and Muscles

With all the hormones produced in your adrenal glands and their regulatory affect on your kidneys and blood pressure, when your adrenal glands become worn-out, your health can suffer major negative impacts. Adrenal fatigue is the term used to describe this condition.

Your adrenal glands are also closely tied to the function of your thyroid. Therefore, any problems in your adrenal glands can result in a strain on your thyroid. This can lead to hypothyroidism and its associate problems, like weight gain, depression, and fatigue.

Ragland's Test – Learn Whether You Are Suffering from Adrenal Fatigue

Ragland's Test is an easy test to perform at home with only a blood pressure cuff. The results of the test are an excellent indicator of whether or not your adrenal glands are working properly. In Ragland's test, you will check your blood pressure while sitting, standing, and lying down.

When you go from lying down to standing, it is the job of your adrenal glands to produce a small amount of the hormone, adrenalin, to help constrict your blood vessels. This tightening of the blood vessels prevents gravity from causing your blood to drop from your head to your feet. If the adrenals aren't able to produce the adrenalin, your blood pressure will drop and you may get a head rush or feel dizzy. Ragland's Test indicates adrenal fatigue when you go from sitting to standing if your systolic pressure does not rise by 4-12 points.

The test indicates a kidney problem if when you go from sitting to lying down, the systolic does not decrease by 4-12 points. As we previously discussed, your kidneys make the chemical messenger renin. Renin, along with hormones produced in your adrenals, affects the tension of your blood vessels, your absorption of sodium, and controls the fluid volume of your blood, all of which regulates your blood pressure. Therefore, a problem in your kidneys can be seen by your body's lack of ability to regulate your blood pressure.

Performing Ragland's Test – Step by Step Instructions

1. Sit comfortably.
2. Using an automatic blood pressure cuff, take a blood pressure reading while you are sitting.
3. Stand up and immediately take your blood pressure again.
4. Chart the two readings in the Workbook section provided.
5. If your blood pressure drops or your systolic pressure does not rise by 4-12 points, you should suspect adrenal fatigue and seek help from a knowledgeable Chiropractic Physician.
6. Lie down on your bed and again take your blood pressure. If your systolic does not decrease by 4-12 points, your test indicates a kidney problem.

Tip: In order to get the most accurate readings possible when performing Ragland's Test, it is better to use an automatic blood pressure cuff rather than a manual one. Due to the changes in the position of your body and the need for immediate readings, manual cuffs simply can't offer quick enough readings.

What to Do If Your Test Results Are Abnormal

Now you understand the importance of your adrenal glands to your blood pressure, kidney and thyroid function, and overall health. If you are suffering from adrenal fatigue, you could have a long list of symptoms which have been negatively impacting your life for months or even years.

If after performing Ragland's Test by following the steps above, you find that your blood pressure drops when you stand up or does not rise by at least 4-12 points or does not drop at least 4-12 points when you lie down, it is time to get help.

A knowledgeable Chiropractic Physician will be able to test you for adrenal fatigue, hormone insufficiencies, nutritional deficiencies, thyroid and kidney issues, dietary problems and much more. This holistic approach will help you find the cause of your adrenal fatigue, correct the problem, resolve the symptoms, and improve your health.

Taking this holistic approach vs. the traditional medicine approach is extremely important to your health in the long run. Unlike the tests and treatment your Chiropractic physician will provide, in the traditional medical approach, adrenal insufficiency is treated with steroids, which have many, often serious side effects.

Side Effects of Steroid Use

Glaucoma	Increased Blood Pressure
Swelling and Fluid Retention	Cataracts
Mood Swings	Weight Gain
High Blood Sugar	Lowered Immune System
Menstrual Irregularities	Calcium Loss From Bones
Easy Bruising	Slow Wound Healing
Increased risk of infection	Malfunctioning adrenal gland

Be sure to notice that one side effect of steroid use is suppressed adrenal gland function, the exact thing the traditional medical doctors are supposed to be treating you for.

Taking into account the list of side effects and the lack of focus on the cause of the adrenal fatigue in the traditional medical system, it is clear that seeking help from a knowledgeable Chiropractic Physician, who will treat the cause, not just the symptoms is the best path to better health.

Your Homework

Now that you understand Ragland's Test and what it tells you about the health of your adrenal system, it is time to check your status.

Your homework for this chapter is to follow the above instructions and perform Ragland's test at home for 3 days. Always chart your results in the Workbook section of the book. This is a written record for both you and your Chiropractic Physician should you need treatment.

What's Next?

In the next chapter, you will learn how to perform the Pin Light Pupillary Test, what the results mean to your health, and when to seek help.

With this chapter, you have taken one more step to regaining control of your health. Congratulate yourself for your dedication.

Chapter 6:

The Pin Light Pupillary Test and Your Adrenal Function

Chapter 6:

The Pin Light Pupillary Test and Your Adrenal Function

As you learned in the previous chapter, your adrenal glands are very important to your overall health and well-being. They make very important hormones, affect your kidneys and your thyroid gland function, and regulate your blood pressure.

When your adrenals are fatigued, you can suffer from many symptoms from mild to severe and debilitating. You will find a list of symptoms in the previous chapter but some of the most common symptoms of adrenal fatigue are sleep problems, overall tiredness, a mental fog, weight gain, depression, low blood pressure, dizziness when you stand, and muscle and joint pain. The list of problems caused by adrenal fatigue is long and involved and shows what a key role these glands play in maintaining your health.

In the last chapter we discussed Ragland's Test, a blood pressure test to help determine whether or not your adrenal glands are compromised. In this chapter you will learn how to perform the Pin Light Pupillary Test, a second test to confirm adrenal fatigue.

Preventive Care Through Home Testing

Questions to Check Your Adrenal Function

To discover whether you are at risk for adrenal fatigue, ask yourself the following questions. If you answer yes to any of these, you may be suffering from adrenal gland suppression:

1. Do you have a hard time falling asleep at night?
2. Do you wake up often during the night?
3. In the morning, do you have a hard time waking up?
4. Do you still feel exhausted after a full night's sleep?
5. Have you gained weight recently without a change in diet or medications?
6. When you stand up, do you feel dizzy or light-headed?
7. Do you feel anxious or stressed?
8. Does bright light bother you more than it should?
9. Have you noticed a change in your food cravings?
10. Are you depressed?
11. Do your feet and hands feel cold?
12. Have you had abdominal pain, nausea, or vomiting?
13. Have you been experiencing constipation?

How the Pin Light Pupillary Test Works

When you are suffering from adrenal fatigue, your eyes are very sensitive to light. This sensitivity is due the fact that when the adrenals are worn-out, the pupils of the eye are unable to constrict correctly.

The Pin Light Pupillary Test primarily tests the adrenal hormone, aldosterone. When aldosterone is low, it causes a decrease of sodium and potassium. This results in the sphincter muscles of your pupils weakening so that they are unable to constrict properly in response to light.[15]

Performing the Pin Light Pupillary Test – Step By Step Instructions

The Pin Light Pupillary Test is a very simple test to perform by yourself at home. All you need for the test is a penlight, or a small flashlight, and a mirror.

1. **Darken the room and allow your eyes to adjust to the light level and get the most accurate results.**
2. **Stand in front of a mirror.**
3. **Place the edge of your hand on the bridge of your nose between your eyes. This blocks the light and allows you to test each eye separately.**
4. **Using a penlight or small flashlight, shine the light into your eye from the side.**
5. **Watch your pupil carefully for 30 seconds.**
6. **In a person without adrenal problems, the pupil will constrict, or get smaller, and stay small as long as the light is shining into it.**

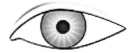

Eye with Pupil Constricted

7. **But, in a person with adrenal fatigue, the pupil will constrict, or get smaller, at first but within 30 seconds, it will dilate, or**

---

[15] Bowthorpe, J, M.Ed. "Stop the Thyroid Madness". 2nd Ed. 2011. Ch.5.

enlarge, again or begin constricting and dilating in a "pulsating" fashion. This is due to a lack of the hormone aldosterone made by the adrenal glands.

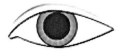

Eye with Pupil Dilated

8. Repeat this procedure on your other eye.
9. Record your results in the Workbook section of this book.

What Your Results Mean

If when you follow the steps above and perform the Pin Light Pupillary Test, and your pupils remain constricted for the 30 seconds, you are unlikely to be suffering from adrenal fatigue.

However, if your pupils contract, get smaller, but then dilate again, or "pulsate" you may have adrenal gland insufficiency. Consider your results together with your results from Ragland's Test, which you performed in the previous chapter. If both tests are positive for adrenal fatigue, there is almost certainly a problem with your adrenals and you should seek care right away.

You may have been suffering for years with chronic fatigue, depression, sleeplessness, weight gain, low blood pressure, low blood sugar, and a host of other problems simply because your adrenal glands were not producing the hormones your body needs to function optimally.

How to Find Help

As you have already learned, it is incredibly important to choose a physician that will take into account all aspects of your health to find the cause of your adrenal insufficiency and not just treat the problem.

Traditional medicine's approach to adrenal insufficiency, as we discussed in the previous chapter, is to use steroids. These result in a long list of side effects, including weight gain, sleeplessness, nervousness, swelling and fluid retention, high blood pressure, easy bruising, and even greater suppression of the adrenal glands. This suppression of adrenal function by the very medicine meant to treat it can lead to a never-ending cycle of decreased adrenal function followed by increasing doses of the prescription. It is a cycle that will only further harm your adrenal system.

Your Chiropractic Physician can take a multi-disciplinary approach to your adrenal fatigue. By checking your hormone levels, diet, exercise, nutrition, vitamins and supplements, stress, fatigue, depression, and much more, they will be able to recommend a comprehensive treatment plan to rev up your adrenals so that you can lead a happier more active life.

Your Homework

In the last two chapters you have learned how to test your adrenal glands, what they mean to your health, and what to do if you find a problem.

Your homework for this chapter is to perform the Pin Light Pupillary Test on both of your eyes and note the results in the Workbook section of the book. Compare the results of this test with the results from the Ragland's test you performed in the previous chapter.

If both tests are normal, your adrenal glands are most likely healthy and working well.

But, if one or both of the tests shows a possibility of adrenal fatigue, seek care with a qualified Chiropractic Physician to get your health back on track as soon as possible.

What's Next?

In the next chapter, you will learn to how to do the Calcium Blood Pressure Cuff Test and what it means to your health.

With every chapter you complete, you get even closer to a healthier life.

Chapter 7:

The Calcium Blood Pressure Cuff Test

Chapter 7:

The Calcium Blood Pressure Cuff Test

Check the Calcium in Your Muscle Tissue

We all know that calcium is important. You hear about taking calcium to prevent osteoporosis. But, calcium plays many more roles than just keeping your bones healthy. It is the most abundant mineral in your entire body. Not only does it help in the development of you bones and teeth, it vital for muscle contraction, cell metabolism and much more.

In this chapter you are going to learn how to perform the Calcium Blood Pressure Cuff Test to check whether or not you have a sufficient level of calcium in your muscles and why this is important to your health.

But, first we're going to look at the function of calcium in your body and why blood tests are insufficient to test your calcium levels.

Why Calcium Is Important to You

Calcium in necessary for healthier, denser bones at any age. It is also vital for making teeth, and to constrict and relax blood vessels, which affects blood pressure. Calcium is a major part blood clotting and needed for muscle contractions and relaxation and nerve stimulation of the heart muscle. Women are especially prone to calcium deficiency due to the hormone changes of pregnancy and menopause.

Symptoms of Calcium Deficiency	
Muscle Aches and Cramps	Back and Neck Pain
Tooth Decay	Bone Pain and Tenderness
Weak or Deformed Bones	Fracture
Brittle Nails	Dry Skin
Poor Posture	Numbness
Poor Appetite	Bruising
PMS	Kidney Stones
Miscarriage	Osteoporosis
Headaches	Heart Disease

Why Blood Tests Aren't Enough

Calcium occurs in different forms throughout your body. It's in your bones, teeth, blood, muscles, and other tissues. When a calcium blood test is performed, it is only measuring the amount of calcium in the blood at that time and it is measuring it as an electrolyte to determine if there is an adequate amount for nerve conduction.

A calcium blood test actually gives very little insight into whether or not you are suffering from a long-term calcium deficiency and whether there is enough calcium in the parts of your body other than your blood.

Because of these inadequacies, it is important to perform a test that checks the calcium levels in other parts of your body such as the Calcium Blood Pressure Cuff Test.

How the Calcium Blood Pressure Cuff Test Works

In order to perform the Calcium Blood Pressure Cuff Test, you will need a manual blood pressure cuff. An automatic cuff will not allow the control necessary for you to perform the test properly.

In this test you will use the blood pressure cuff around your calf, rather than your arm. You will not need a stethoscope for this test. You will be checking for signs of your calf muscle cramping, not listening for your pulse.

Whether you feel cramping or not and how quickly is an excellent indicator of whether or not your muscles are calcium deficient and whether you should seek care.

Performing the Test – Step By Step Instructions

1. Lie on you back.
2. Bend the knee of the leg you will be checking and put your foot flat on the floor.
3. Strap the blood pressure cuff around your calf. The bottom of the cuff should be about 1 inch above your ankle.
4. Tighten the valve by turning the silver knob so that no air leaks out.
5. Slowly inflate the cuff.
6. Watch for any signs of muscle cramping, even just a twinge.
7. If you are not experiencing cramps, continue to inflate the cuff to 220 mm or slightly higher if tolerated.
8. It is normal to feel a tight pressure. Make sure to distinguish this from actual cramping.
9. Deflate the cuff.

10. Record your findings in the Workbook section of the book.
11. Repeat the procedure on the opposite leg.

What Your Results Mean

If you are able to inflate the blood pressure cuff to 220 mm without cramping, your calcium level in your muscles is normal.

If you experience cramping between 180-220 mm then your calcium level is borderline low and you should seek further testing and treatment.

If your muscles cramped before reaching 180 mm, your calcium level is definitely low and you will need to see a knowledgeable physician who can find the cause of your calcium deficiency.[16]

Warning: This test should not be performed if you have vascular disease.

Differences of Results Between Legs

It is also important to note any difference in cramping between your right and left legs. If you experience cramping in one side

---

[16] Mincin, K, Clin. Nut. "2006" Calcium quick test. Retrieved May 15, 2012 from Nutrition Testing.com www.nutrition-testing.com/nutritionresource/testing1.htm

but not the other or more severe cramping in one it could be a sign of peripheral vascular problems.

It is important that if you have any disparity between sides that you seek the care of a physician knowledgeable in the cause and treatment of these conditions.

How to Find Care

As you now know, calcium affects more than just your bones. It helps your heart to beat. It makes sure your blood vessels dilate and constrict. And, it allows your muscles to contract and relax.

Despite the fact that it is the most abundant nutrient in the human body, many people can suffer from calcium deficiency, sometimes severe.

If after following the steps above, the results of your Calcium Blood Pressure Cuff Test are abnormal, it is time to seek care. Calcium deficiency does not go away on its own and there can be underlying causes, such as Vitamin D deficiency and parathyroid conditions that are important to address promptly.

With the role calcium plays throughout your body, it is more important than ever to choose the care of a Chiropractic Physician who is trained to diagnose and treat the body as a whole. They will check your muscular system, cardiovascular system, hormone levels, vitamin and nutrient deficiencies, and much more to find the underlying cause of your calcium deficiency before it progresses to a serious, symptomatic problem.

Your Homework

Now that you understand the significance calcium has in your health and the functions of your bones, muscles, and organs, you are ready to check your own calcium level.

Follow the above instructions to perform the Calcium Blood Pressure Cuff test. Record your results in the Workbook section provided and seek care when indicated.

Remember, if you feel any cramping between 180-200 mm, your calcium is already dropping. If you have cramping below 180 mm, the calcium in your muscles is very low. In both cases find a knowledgeable Chiropractic Physician for immediate care.

What's Next?

In the next chapter, you will learn how to perform the Broda Barnes Basal Temperature Test, what the test means for both men and women, and how it can be used to assess fertility.

Good health is a journey, not a destination. You are on that journey right now.

Chapter 8:

The Broda Barnes Basal Temperature Test – Thyroid Function and Fertility

Chapter 8:

The Broda Barnes Basal Temperature Test – Thyroid Function and Fertility

Your body temperature is a good indicator of a number of aspects of your health. In this chapter, you will learn how to perform the Broda Barnes Basal Temperature Test to determine whether or not your thyroid gland is functioning optimally. You will also discover how the test can be used to indicate a woman's fertility, even pinpointing ovulation.

Your Thyroid Gland and Your Body Temperature

Your thyroid gland controls your body's metabolic rate, the speed at which every cell in your body burns energy. In this way, your thyroid's function directly influences your body temperature. If your thyroid function is low, your metabolic rate is lowered as is your body temperature. Because of this relationship, your body temperature is a good indicator of whether or not your thyroid is working well.

Traditional medicine uses a blood test to check for thyroid problems. However, blood tests are not sensitive enough to show a moderate thyroid deficiency and usually only indicates a problem when thyroid levels are extremely low. [17]

The Broda Barnes Basal Temperature Test – Step By Step Instructions

The Broda Barnes Basal Temperature Test is a simple test that you can do at home to check your thyroid function. The only thing you need to perform the test is a basal thermometer. This is an axillary (armpit) thermometer that measures your body temperature in tenths of degrees.

1. Place your basal thermometer beside your bed, within reach, before going to sleep.
2. In the morning, before getting out of bed, put the thermometer under your arm, with the bulb in your armpit. There should be no clothing between the bulb and your armpit.
3. Make sure to take your temperature before performing any activity at all. Don't even sit up. Even slight activity will alter your body temperature.
4. The test should be performed at the same time each day. Set an alarm if you need to. A difference of more

---

[17] Sklovsky, R. Pharm. D, ND, PC. "2003" Low thyroid: the unsuspected illness. Retrieved May 15, 2012 from Dr. Bob ND.com www.drbobnd.com/low_thyroid.htm

than 30 minutes between tests can result in inaccurate assessment.

5. Leave the thermometer under your arm for 10 minutes.
6. After 10 minutes, remove the thermometer and check your reading.
7. Immediately record your reading in the Workbook section of this book.
8. For men and women who do not have menstrual cycles, repeat this procedure for 10 days.
9. If you are female, your menstrual cycle will affect your body temperature. Therefore, the test should be done for 30 days or a full cycle. For the convenience of charting, it is best to start on Day 1 of your cycle.

What Your Results Tell You about Your Thyroid

Normal basal body temperature is between 97.8 and 98.2 degrees Fahrenheit (36.6-36.8 degrees Celsius). If your reading is within these limits, your thyroid is functioning normally.

Anything reading below 97.8 F (36.6 C) is considered low and an indication of low thyroid function. While a reading above 98.2F (36.8 C) could indicate an overactive thyroid, a high reading can also indicate infection and fever.

Finding Help If Your Results are Abnormal

Any abnormal readings are an indication of possible problems with your thyroid gland function and you should seek appropriate care to address the cause of the problem. A Chiropractic Physician, knowledgeable in treating all aspect of your health, will be able to analyze your thyroid function and find the cause of any abnormalities. Your Chiropractic Physician can also recommend appropriate treatments, including dietary changes, supplementation, exercise, and more to reverse your thyroid problems and prevent it from causing serious health issues.

The Broda Barnes Basal Temperature Test and Fertility

A woman's basal body temperature increases with an increase of progesterone, a hormone that is released during ovulation that stimulates a warmer environment for a possible developing fetus. Because of this relationship between ovulation and body temperature, the Broda Barnes Basal Temperature Test can also be used to check your fertility, track your ovulation, and increase your chances of becoming pregnant.

Starting on Day One of your menstrual cycle, perform the Broda Barnes Basal Temperature Test every morning, following the step by step instructions above. However, be sure to start on Day One of your cycle rather than Day Three to monitor your fertility rather than your thyroid function. Also, make sure that you take your temperature before getting out of bed, prior to any activity, in order to get an accurate reading.

Due to the release of progesterone during ovulation, your body temperature will rise by a minimum of 0.4 degrees Fahrenheit. By charting the pattern of your daily temperature changes throughout the month, you will be able to pinpoint ovulation, your peak time for conceiving a baby.

Plot your temperature on the chart in the Workbook section of this book every day. When you experience a temperature shift of at least 0.4 F over a 48 hour period, this signals that you are ovulating. The shift should be above your highest temperature in the previous six days. This helps you determine your window of opportunity for becoming pregnant.

If your temperature remains up for 18 days or more following ovulation, you should check for pregnancy. By charting your basal body temperature, you can take greater control over your own fertility and improve your chances of conception.

Monitoring your fertility can also help you keep track of the health of your reproductive system. Changes in your cycle can alert you to potential gynecological problems so that you can seek care before they become serious and symptomatic.

If your Basal Body Temperature chart indicates any changes in your cycle, it is important to find treatment from a Chiropractic Physician who is knowledgeable in all areas of health. Your Chiropractic Physician can analyze possible hormonal changes and determine their underlying cause. They can also recommend appropriate follow-up treatment to ensure that your reproductive system is functioning optimally.

Your Homework

In this chapter, you have learned what clues your body temperature can give you about the health of your thyroid gland and the female reproductive system and fertility.

Your homework for this chapter is to perform the Broda Barnes Basal Body Temperature Test. Men and women who do not have menstrual cycles should perform the test for 10 days. Women with menstrual cycles should perform the test for 30 days or a full cycle. For convenience it is best to start from Day 1 of your cycle. Chart your results in the Workbook section of the book. If your results indicate problems in your thyroid function, you now know how to find the appropriate care to address the problem and prevent serious health concerns.

If you are a woman who is concerned about her fertility or you want to become pregnant, use the Basal Body Temperature Chart in the Workbook section to chart your body temperature to learn more about your reproductive system, discover when you ovulate, and improve your chances of pregnancy.

What's Next?

In the next chapter, you will learn why iodine is important to your health and how to easily test for iodine deficiency at home.

Your health is a choice you make every day. Every time you choose to learn how to protect your health, you increase the quality of your life.

Chapter 9:

The Importance of Iodine for Your Health

Chapter 9:

The Importance of Iodine for Your Health

You have probably heard of iodine before. You've most likely even bought it at the grocery store in the form of iodized salt. But, most people don't know how important iodine is to staying healthy.

In this chapter, you will learn how iodine works in your body, what can happen if you don't have enough, and how to test your iodine levels to avoid deficiency.

What is Iodine and Where Does It Come From?

Iodine is a trace mineral that is naturally found in your body. You can get iodine through iodized salt (table salt with iodine added to it), sea salt, seafood like cod, haddock, and seabass, eggs, and dairy products, like cheese and yogurt. But, the best source of iodine is kelp, a sea vegetable.

Vegetables, like onions and radishes, can also contain iodine if the soil they are grown in has iodine in it. Unfortunately, there is less iodine in our soil every year due to the chemicals used to prevent pests and disease and the over-use of the soil. Now, the soil that our vegetables are grown in is mostly over-worked, worn out, and depleted of nutrients.

The soil in the Midwest is especially iodine deficient. Because of this, the food grown here is extremely deficient in iodine. In fact, due to this iodine deficiency and the incidence of goiters from thyroid problems, the Midwest is known as the "goiter belt".

Are You Getting Enough Iodine in Your Diet?

Iodine deficiency is becoming more and more common. Women are especially prone to this deficiency due to the fact that a woman's thyroid gland is twice as large as the thyroid gland in men. Since the thyroid is the main consumer of iodine in the body, women will normally require more iodine than men to stay healthy. This need increases even more with pregnancy.

In 1940, the typical American consumed approximately 800 micrograms of iodine every day. By 1995, that number had plummeted to only 135 micrograms, an 83% drop.[18]

---

[18]Alternative Medicine Angel. "2000" How to self test for iodine deficiency. Retrieved on May 15, 2012 from Altmedangel.com http://altmedangel.com/iodine.htm

If you eat a typical American diet, it is very likely that you are not getting enough iodine each day and will suffer form iodine deficiency at some point in your life.

Iodine and Your Thyroid Gland

Your thyroid gland is in the lower, front part of your neck and sits across your trachea, or windpipe. It is responsible for your body's metabolism (how fast you burn calories). It also controls your body's sensitivity to other hormones and dictates how hormones are produced.

The major job of your thyroid gland is to produce thyroid hormone. Thyroid hormone helps your body make energy, regulates your body temperature, and helps your other organs function properly.

Your thyroid makes two major hormones, triiodothyronine, called T3, and thyroxine, called T4. The 3 and 4 refer to the number of iodine molecules needed to make these hormones.

Iodine combines with tyrosine, an amino acid to form these hormones. So, three iodine molecules plus tyrosine make T3, or triiodothyronine. And, 4 iodine molecules plus tyrosine make T4, or thyroxine.

A healthy thyroid will produces approximately 20% T3 and 80% T4. In order to make these hormones, your thyroid gland uses two-thirds of the iodine in your body, making iodine absolutely essential to a healthy, fully-functioning thyroid.

Without enough iodine, the thyroid can't make its hormones. Your thyroid stops functioning properly. This is known as hypothyroidism and there are many symptoms associated with it, some severe. Some of the most common problems you experience with hypothyroidism are that your metabolism slows down, your other organs and your body as a whole don't function as well, you feel tired and sluggish, you may gain weight, and it can be hard to think clearly.

Symptoms of Hypothyrodism[19]

Fatigue	Mental Fog
Weakness	Irritability
Weight Gain	Constipation
Difficulty Losing Weight	Abnormal Menstrual Cycle
Hair Loss	Decreased Libido
Dry, Brittle Hair	Fertility Problems
Dry, Flaky Skin	Low Body Temperature
Sensitivity to Cold	Swollen Thyroid Gland or Goiter
Muscle Cramps	Hoarse, Gravelly Voice
Depression	Memory Loss

---

[19] Goodson, D. "2005" What are the symptoms of hypothyroidism. Retrieved May 15, 2012 from A 2 Z of Health, Beauty, and Fitness Health.learninginfo.org/hypothyroidism.htm

If you don't have enough iodine in your diet, you can even end

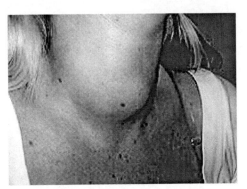

up with a goiter, an abnormally swollen thyroid gland that can cause a large swelling of your neck. Untreated, goiters can be permanent and worsen.

A small goiter can be seen in this woman's neck (above).

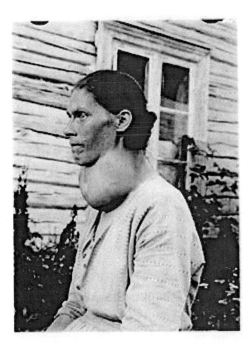

This woman's goiter (left) has obviously been untreated and progressed for many years.

Other than the creation of the thyroid hormones, iodine is also needed by the thyroid to prevent the build-up of toxic chemicals in the gland. Iodine helps to clear them out of the thyroid and in iodine deficiency, environmental pollutants, like fluoride, can accumulate inside of the gland and block its normal function.

With all of the important processes iodine is used for by your thyroid gland, it is easy to see that getting enough iodine in your diet is essential to the healthy functioning of your thyroid. But, that is not all iodine does. It is also necessary for many of your other body functions.

How Iodine Is Used In the Rest of Your Body

Iodine is used by every gland and mucosal lining in your body. It is essential for cell metabolism and also helps your body's hormone receptors function properly so that your hormones can communicate more efficiently with your organs.

Iodine acts as a buffer against estrogen and is needed in high concentrations in the both the ovaries and the breasts. When a woman has enough iodine in these tissues, her female sex hormones will perform better.

The breasts and the prostate gland are the second largest storage site for iodine, following the thyroid gland. Iodine is also used by your adrenal glands, your parotid glands, and in the mucosal lining of your intestines.

Even more important, iodine is crucial for brain function and intelligence. Many studies have shown the importance of iodine during pregnancy, both to help the mother's thyroid gland and for the development of the baby's brain.

Testing for Iodine Deficiency at Home

Since having enough iodine in your body is vital to so many of your body's organs and functions, including those of your thyroid gland and brain, knowing whether or not you are deficient in iodine can save you from many health problems.

The Iodine Skin Test is an easy way to determine if you are suffering from an iodine deficiency that could be negatively impacting your health. To perform the test, all you need is a liquid tincture of 2% iodine, found at your local pharmacy, and a cotton swab.

Iodine Skin Test – Step By Step Instructions

1. Wipe your body dry after a bath or shower.
2. Using a cotton swab, apply the iodine solution on your inner thigh or upper arm.
3. Paint the area to cover a 2 inch diameter, or the size of a silver dollar.
4. Don't put any lotions, creams, or deodorants on the area.
5. Allow the area to remain untouched and check it after 8 hours, 12 hours, and 24 hours.
6. Chart the results in the Workbook section of this book.

Interpreting Your Results

If the iodine patch disappears within 8 hours, you are very deficient in iodine. If the patch is gone prior to the 12 hour mark, your iodine level is low and will need to be addressed. In both cases, you should seek the care of a knowledgeable professional to help you determine the cause of the deficiency and suggest proper supplementation.

If after 24 hours, your iodine patch has still not gone away, you are not iodine deficient. Continue to perform the Iodine Skin Test on a monthly basis to ensure that your iodine levels remain normal.

How to Find Help if You Are Iodine Deficient

If your test results indicate that your iodine levels are low, it is vital that you seek the care of a Chiropractic Physician who can analyze the results of your test, check the functioning of your thyroid gland, assess your hormone levels, and find the cause of your iodine deficiency. Your Chiropractic Physician can also suggest appropriate iodine supplementation to improve your health and prevent the deficiency from progressing.

Your Homework

Now that you have learned the important role iodine plays in the health of your thyroid gland and other organs of your body and the severe symptoms you can suffer when you do not have enough iodine in your diet, it is time to test your iodine levels at home.

Your homework for this chapter is to perform the Iodine Skin Test and record the results in the Workbook section. If your iodine patch does not disappear within 24 hours, your iodine levels are normal. Simply continue to do the test on a monthly basis as a health check.

If your patch disappeared prior to the 24 hour time period, by the 8 or 12 hour mark, you are iodine deficient and it is time to get help. Just by not having enough iodine for your body to work properly, you may have been suffering from chronic symptoms like fatigue, weight gain, depression, and much more.

What's Next?

In the next chapter, you will find out how zinc affects your health and how to easily check your levels, just by looking at your fingernails.

With each chapter you read, you learn more about your body, giving you the power to make the best decisions possible about your healthcare.

Chapter 10:

The Zinc Nail Test — How Your Fingernails Warn You of Zinc Deficiency

Chapter 10:

The Zinc Nail Test – How Your Fingernails Warn You of Zinc Deficiency

Zinc is an essential trace element. It is crucial for your immune system, brain function, growth, development, and fertility. Yet, many people are living without enough zinc in their bodies to function normally. The longer you remain deficient in zinc, the more your health deteriorates.

Fortunately, there is an easy test that you can do at home to check whether or not you are getting enough zinc. The best part is that it just requires you to look at your fingernails.

In this chapter, you will learn why zinc is important to your body, where zinc comes from, what can happen to you if you don't get enough, and how to do the Zinc Nail Test to check your own zinc levels.

Why Zinc Is Important to You

Zinc is one of the most important of all trace elements for your body. It is essential for the proper function of cellular metabolism. It helps your immune system, protects your cell membranes from damage, controls the release of hormones, and the transmission of nerve impulses. It helps in cell reproduction and wound healing and plays a vital role in fertility and conception.

By binding to DNA and helping the genes tell cells what to do, including when to die, zinc can play an important role in the prevention of cancer. Zinc is one of nature's strongest antioxidants. It also helps to protect the liver, detoxify alcohol, and helps in the storage of insulin in your body. More than 100 specific enzymes require zinc for their function.[20]

Dietary Sources of Zinc

Zinc occurs in a variety of food but is most common in animal sources or proteins, especially beef, pork, chicken, fish, oysters, and even eggs and dairy products. It can also be found in lesser amounts in nuts, seeds, beans, and mushrooms. Brewer's Yeast, a whole-grain product that you can add to other foods, is also a good source of zinc. It can be found at your local health food store or most vitamin stores.

---

[20] Cousins, RI. Zinc. In: Present Knowledge in Nutrition. Ed. Zeigler EE, Filer LJ. Washington DC. ILSI Press 1996.

Causes of Zinc Deficiency

Conservative estimates are that at least 25% of our population is at risk for zinc deficiency.[21] It is the fifth leading risk factor for disease in the developed world. Zinc deficiency is primarily caused by a shortage of dietary zinc.

It has been found that people that consume primarily plant based diets, especially vegetarians, have a much higher risk of zinc deficiency than people who consume a primarily protein based diet. The typical American diet, containing processed food, very little protein, and vegetables grown in nutrient-depleted soil offers very little zinc.

In fact, according to Ananda S. Prasad, MD, PhD, of Wayne State University, "The Western world's shift from consumption of meat proteins to cereal proteins may precipitate a general increase in zinc deficiency."[22]

Even worse, because your body can only absorb approximately 30% of the zinc you take in, zinc deficiency can easily happen to you.

Other than nutritional shortage, zinc deficiency can also be caused by pregnancy, surgery, malabsorption, excessive alcohol

---

[21] Sandstead, MW. (2006). "Zinc requirements and the risks and benefits of zinc supplementation". *J Trace Elem Med Biol* **20** (1): 3–18.

[22] Eby, G. "2011" Warning! Zinc deficiency—as cause of modern illnesses. Retrieved May 16, 2012 from George Eby Research Institute http://george-eby-research.com/html/warning.html

use, fasting, chronic liver or kidney disease, diabetes, environmental toxins, cancer, and other chronic illnesses.

Zinc deficiency is most common in women, children, and the elderly but can happen to anyone.

Symptoms of Zinc Deficiency

Since zinc has so many functions in your body, a lack of it can lead to many symptoms. And, long periods of zinc deficiency can result in severe trouble for your health. Zinc is in fact so important to the body's health that tests in animals have shown that a zinc deficiency resulted in immune system depression not only in the specific animal, but also in their children, all the way to the third generation.[23]

Smoking in combination with zinc deficiency leads to even worse health problems. Since smoking tobacco allows zinc to be replaced by cadmium, which is toxic to the body, this combination results in lung disease.

---

[23] "Gestational zinc deprivation in mice: persistence of immunodeficiency for three generations". Science. 1982, Vol. 218. 469-471.

Signs and Symptoms of Zinc Deficiency[24]

White Spots on the Fingernails	Skin Rashes
Impaired Sense of Taste and Smell	Anorexia
Poor Hair Growth	Hair Loss
Depression	Irritability
Mental Illness	Lethargy
Poor Growth in Children	Infertility
Slow Wound Healing	Acne
Diarrhea	Memory Loss
Pneumonia	Dysmenorrhea
Lowered Immune System	Asthma
Poor Appetite	Vision Problems
Free Radical Damage	Frequent Infections
Premature Aging	Loss of Hair Color
Stretch Marks	Joint Pain
Cognitive Impairment	Birth Defects

Checking for Zinc Deficiency at Home

Zinc deficiency is a serious health problem and you could be at risk. It is very important that you know whether or not you are getting enough zinc to support a healthy body so that you can prevent disease and seek proper care when necessary.

---

[24] Office of Dietary Supplement. "2011" Dietary supplement fact sheet: zinc". Retrieved May 15, 2012 from National Institute of Health ods.od.nih.gov/factsheets/zinc-HealthProfessional/

Preventive Care Through Home Testing

The Zinc Nail Test is an easy way to check for zinc deficiency in your own home and no equipment is needed. Since zinc deficiency often causes white spots on the fingernails, you can look for signs of the problem just by examining your own fingernails.

Performing the Zinc Nail Test – Step By Step Instructions

1. In a room with good light, observe your fingernails.
2. Look for white spots, lines, or bands.

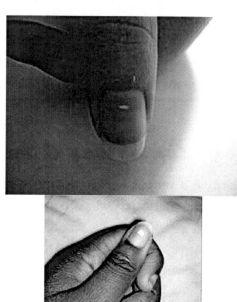

3. Record your results in the Workbook section of the book.

4. We recommend that you take a picture of any fingernails with white spots. If you are unable to get a photograph of them, draw a picture in the provided space in the Workbook to show how many spots, lines, or bands there are and their location on the nail.

Interpreting Your Results

Any white spots on your fingernails can be a sign of zinc deficiency and you should seek help from a knowledgeable Physician who can analyze your zinc status, find the cause of any deficiency, and set up a treatment plan to correct it.

Some women may even notice parallel white lines on their fingernails. These lines indicate repeated zinc deficiency during their menstrual cycles.

How to Find Treatment if You Suspect Zinc Deficiency

If your fingernails showed white spots, bands, or lines, you should suspect zinc deficiency. Since any zinc deficiency can lead to a multitude of health problems, it is imperative that you seek the care of a Chiropractic Physician who will determine if you are zinc deficient and find the cause behind your deficiency. Your Chiropractic Physician will analyze your diet, nutrition, supplements, chronic health problems, and many more factors to establish the cause of the deficiency.

They will also be able to set up an appropriate treatment plan to reverse the deficiency and prevent the health complications it causes from becoming serious and symptomatic. This treatment plan could include dietary changes, supplementation, addressing other health problems, such as malabsorption, and more.

Your Homework

In this chapter, you learned why zinc is so important to your body and what can happen to your health if you are not getting enough zinc in your diet or are unable to utilize it due to other disease processes.

Your homework for this chapter is to perform the Zinc Nail Test. Check your fingernails for white spots, bands, or lines and record your results in the Workbook section of the book. If possible, take a picture of any fingernails that are abnormal or draw picture of them in the Workbook.

If you find signs of zinc deficiency, it is time to seek help to find the cause of the problem and reverse the deficiency before the impact on your health worsens.

What's Next?

In the next chapter, you will learn how to perform the Zinc Oral Solution Test to confirm zinc deficiency. This test together with the Zinc Nail Test you learned in this chapter offer an excellent way to check your zinc levels and needs.

Each change you make to improve your health makes a positive impact on your life.

Chapter 11:

Zinc Oral Solution Test – Confirming Zinc Deficiency

Chapter 11:

Zinc Oral Solution Test – Confirming Zinc Deficiency

As you learned in the previous chapter, zinc is one of the most important trace elements in the body. Zinc supports proper growth and development during pregnancy, childhood, and adolescence.[25] It is vital for cellular metabolism, supports your immune system, helps in wound healing, and much more. Yet, with all of the needs the body has for zinc, it doesn't have a way to store the zinc it needs. This means that a regular daily intake of zinc is required to maintain your health.[26]

The Importance of Zinc to Your Health

Zinc performs so many vital functions in your body. Yet, due to poor diet, malabsorption, and the nutrient depletion of our soil, more and more people in our country are at risk for zinc

---

[25] Simmer K, Thompson RP. Zinc in the fetus and newborn. Acta Paediatr Scand Suppl 1985;319:158-63. [HPubMed abstractH]
[26] Rink L, Gabriel P. Zinc and the immune system. Proc Nutr Soc 2000;59:541-52. [HPubMed abstractH]

deficiency every day, causing an increase of its associated health problems.

Functions of Zinc

- Helps Prevent Cancer
- Antioxidant
- Detoxification of the Liver
- Collagen Synthesis
- Essential for Fertility
- Protects the Immune System
- Necessary for the Storage of Insulin
- Wound Healing
- Required for more than 100 enzyme activities
- Controls the Release of Hormones
- Helps in the Transportation of Carbon Dioxide
- Helps Nerve Impulse Transmission
- Helps Prevent Blindness
- Associated With Aging
- Crucial for the Structure and Function of the Cell Membrane

Dr. Vladimir Gordin

What Puts You at Risk for Zinc Deficiency?

There are many risk factors for zinc deficiency but the most likely cause is eating the typical American diet. With more processed foods, and less proteins in your diet, your risk of zinc deficiency goes up substantially.

Other risk factors include problems with absorption, such as gastrointestinal problems, pregnancy, eating a vegetarian diet, overuse of alcohol, and chronic liver and kidney disease.

Health Problems Associated With Zinc Deficiency

Zinc deficiency decreases immune function, slows wound healing, and increases your susceptibility to infections, like pneumonia.[27] Zinc has even been used to reduce the severity and duration of the common cold by inhibiting the rhinovirus and suppressing inflammation.[28]

Zinc deficiency has been linked to diarrhea, vision loss, anorexia, cognitive and motor function impairment, growth failures, like dwarfism, fertility problems, and free radical damage.

---

[27] Shankar AH, Prasad AS. Zinc and immune function: the biological basis of altered resistance to infection. Am J Clin Nutr 1998;68:447S-63S.

[28] Hulisz D. Efficacy of zinc against common cold viruses: an overview. J Am Pharm Assoc (2003) 2004;44:594-603.

Home Testing for Zinc Deficiency

In the last chapter, you learned how to perform the Zinc Nail Test to check for white spots, bands, or lines on your fingernails that can indicate that you are deficient in zinc. There is one more test that is easy to do at home and is helpful in determining whether you are lacking zinc. It is called the Zinc Oral Solution Test. The results of these two tests taken together give you excellent feedback on your body's need for zinc and the possible health problems you could be at risk for due to zinc deficiency.

Because your senses of taste and smell are dependent upon their being enough zinc in your body, you can establish your zinc status by using a standard test solution of zinc sulfate for tasting and comparing your response to certain defined standards. Zinc Oral Tests can easily be ordered online. They are simply a combination of zinc sulfate, elemental zinc, and purified water. The concentration of the zinc sulfate to purified water is 1 gram per liter. The liquid can be kept refrigerated after opening for up to six months.

The Zinc Oral Solution Test – Step by Step Instructions

1. Do not eat, drink, or smoke for at least one hour prior to the test.

2. Hold 10 ml (2 tsp.) of the Zinc Solution in your mouth for 10 seconds. Then, you can spit it out.

3. Rate your taste or sensation based on the standards listed below.

4. Record your results in the Workbook section of this book.

Your Results and What They Mean

1. If you have no specific taste sensation with from the Zinc Oral Solution, it just tastes like plain water; this indicates a major zinc deficiency.

2. If you don't notice a taste immediately but within the ten seconds of the test, a dry or metallic taste is experienced, this indicates a moderate zinc deficiency.

3. If you notice an immediate, slight taste that is not necessarily unpleasant but builds over the 10 second time period, this indicates a minor zinc deficiency.

4. If you notice an immediate, strong, unpleasant taste from the solution, this indicates that you are not zinc deficient.

Tip: If you have a number of amalgam fillings in your teeth, the Zinc Oral Solution Test may be less precise. The mixture of the zinc solution plus the mercury from the amalgams can cause a strong, metallic taste in your mouth even if you are severely zinc deficient.

How to Find Care for Your Zinc Deficiency

If the results of your Zinc Oral Solution Test fell into any of the first 3 categories, it indicates that you are suffering from a zinc deficiency that needs to be addressed. Combined with the results of your Zinc Nail Test from the previous chapter, you now have a very good indication of your zinc status.

With the importance of zinc to maintaining a healthy body, it is critical that you seek the care of a Chiropractic Physician knowledgeable in treating all aspects of the human body to find the cause of your zinc deficiency and recommend appropriate treatment, including dietary changes, supplementation, and much more.

Your Homework

With a thorough understanding of how zinc works in your body and why it is so vital to your health, you are now prepared to check your own zinc status.

Your homework for this chapter is to perform the Zinc Oral Solution Test, grade your results based on the standards listed above, and record the results in your Workbook section. If your results indicate a zinc deficiency, you now know how to find appropriate care for your condition.

If both the Zinc Oral Solution Test and the Zinc Nail Test from the previous chapter indicate no zinc deficiency, then you are already on the path to good health. Continue to perform both tests once a month to keep track of your zinc status and prevent disease.

What's Next?

In the next chapter, you will learn how Candida affects your life and your health and how to determine if your wellbeing may be negatively impacted by this problem.

Small steps toward better health lead to a huge improvement in the quality of your life.

Chapter 12:

The Candida Spit Test – Candida Overgrowth and the Danger to Your Health

Chapter 12:

The Candida Spit Test – Candida Overgrowth and the Danger to Your Health

Candida Albicans is the most common type of yeast in your body. It lives in your mucous membranes and your skin. When your body is healthy and in balance, Candida doesn't cause any issues. But, when the balance of Candida to other bacteria shifts, you can end up with serious health problems.

In this chapter, you will learn what Candida is, the dangers to your health caused by Candida overgrowth, and how to perform the Candida Spit Test to check the level of Candida in your body at home.

What is Candida?

Candida is a yeast or fungus that is normally found in the digestive system, mouth, vagina, penis, and rectum. Under normal circumstances, the Candida in your body is controlled by the beneficial bacteria that also live in balance with it. However, if the bacteria-Candida balance is upset, Candida overgrowth, or Candidiasis is the result.

Candidiasis and Dysbacteriosis

Dysbacteriosis is condition where the flora in your body's intestinal tract is altered. After birth, your intestines become colonized by many different kinds of bacteria.[29] These beneficial bacteria help your body to absorb vitamins and minerals and keep dangerous organisms and fungus from flourishing.

When the healthy bacteria is killed or suppressed, you are pushed into a state of dysbacteriosis. The loss of the beneficial bacteria allows yeasts, like Candida, to thrive and grow and Candidiasis is the consequence. The Candida feeds on the foods you eat and produces its own waste products. These waste products are toxic to your system and result in numerous health problems.

---

[29] Intestinal Dysbiosis. "2011" Intestinal dysbiosis: my story. Retrieved May 16, 2012 from Intestinal Dysbiosis.com http://intestinaldysbiosis.com/dysbiosis/dysbacteriosis-symptoms-treatment

Causes of Candida Overgrowth

There are a number of things that can lead to the suppression of the beneficial bacteria in your body, allowing Candida to grow unchecked.

The primary cause of Candidiasis is antibiotic treatment. Antibiotics are not targeted to just destroy bad bacteria. They kill both beneficial and harmful bacteria.

When your beneficial bacteria are destroyed, Candida will grow unimpeded.

Unfortunately, many people take multiple antibiotics every year, each time destroying more beneficial bacteria and each time allowing more Candida to take over their body and ruin their health.

The typical American diet of refined, processed, sugary foods is also a leading cause of Candida overgrowth.

Candida feeds on the sugar and starches in your system.

And, the usual refined foods eaten every day in our country provide an abundance of these sugars for the Candida in your body to use and grow.

Foods that support your body's beneficial bacteria are also sadly lacking in this type of diet. Fermented dairy products supply a source of this necessary bacteria.

But, few people consume enough of it to promote a healthy balance of bacteria to Candida in their system.

Alcoholism and a suppressed immune system also create an environment where Candida thrives.

Effects of Candidiasis on Your Health

Once the balance between the beneficial bacteria and the Candida in your system is disrupted and the Candida begins to grow, your health suffers.

The Candida and its waste products slip into your blood stream, finding their way to all parts of your body.

This can lead to joint and organ problems, sinusitis, and much more.

It also covers your intestinal walls, interfering with the digestion of your food and blocking the absorption of nutrients.

This can cause bloating, constipation, gas, diarrhea, food allergies, and many other digestive issues.[30]

---

[30] Lipschultz-Robinson, S. "1996" Candida: conquering yeast infections – the non-drug solution. Retrieved on May 16, 2012 from Shirley's Wellness Café http://www.shirleys-wellness-cafe.com/candida.htm

Symptoms of Candidiasis	
Vaginal Itching/Burning	Vaginal Discharge
Lowered Immune System	Vaginal Odor
Painful Sex	Fatigue
Menstrual Pain	Urinary Difficulties
Irritability	PMS
Impotence	Poor Memory
Digestive Pain	Constipation
Depression	Gas
Bloating	Short Attention Span
Joint Pain/Swelling	Arthritis
Shortness of Breath	Muscle Aches
Headaches	Thrush
Respiratory Infections	Food Allergies
Learning Problems	Low Blood Sugar
Acne	Skin Rashes

Are You Suffering From Candidiasis?

You may be experiencing many of the above symptoms due to an overgrowth of Candida in your system. Or, you may have too much Candida in your body but have not yet felt the outward effects. Either way, you must find out if your system is out of balance so that you can find the appropriate care to treat the problem before it leads to serious health issues.

Preventive Care Through Home Testing

If you are wondering if Candida is negatively impacting your health, complete the following questionnaire, created by Dr. William G. Crook, in his book, "The Yeast Connection: A Medical Breakthrough".[31]

If you answer "yes" to any question, check it and add up your score.

1. Have you taken repeated or prolonged courses of antibiotics?   Yes   4
2. Do you have recurrent vaginal, prostate, or urinary infections?   Yes   3
3. Do you feel "sick" all over but no cause has been found?   Yes   2
4. Do you have PMS, menstrual problems, sexual dysfunction, sugar cravings, low body temperature, or fatigue?   Yes   2
5. Are you sensitive to tobacco smoke, perfumes, or other odors?   Yes   2
6. Do you have memory or concentration problems?   Yes   2
7. Have you taken prolonged courses of steroids, or birth control?   Yes   2
8. Do some foods cause you problems or trigger symptoms?   Yes   1
9. Do you have constipation, diarrhea, bloating, or abdominal pain? Yes   1
10. Does your skin itch, tingle, or burn, is dry, or has rashes?   Yes   1

---

[31] Crook, W, MD. "The Yeast Connection: A Medical Breakthrough". Vintage Books. 1986.

Scoring for Women: If your score is 9 or more, your health problems are probably related to Candida. With a score of 12 or more, your health problems are definitely related to Candida.

Scoring for Men: If your score is 7 or more, your health problems are probably related to Candida. With a score of 10 or more, your health problems are definitely related to Candida.

After checking your score, it is important to perform the Candida Spit Test to verify whether you are suffering from Candida overgrowth.

The Candida Spit Test - Step By Step Instructions

The Candida Spit (Saliva) Test is a very simple procedure that you can perform at home with only a glass of water to determine if the Candida in your body is out of balance with your beneficial bacteria.

1. Perform this test as soon as you wake up in the morning, before putting anything into your mouth.
2. Fill a clear glass with room-temperature, bottled water.
3. Spit into the glass of water.
4. Check the water every 15 minutes for 1 hour.
5. If you have potential problems with Candidiasis, you will see strings, like legs, threading down into the water.
6. Candida overgrowth is also indicated if "cloudy" saliva sinks to the bottom of the glass or cloudy specks are seen suspended in the water.

SALIVA TEST

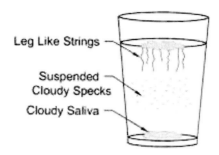

Leg Like Strings

Suspended
Cloudy Specks

Cloudy Saliva

7. If you see no strings and your saliva is still floating on top of the water after one hour, Candida overgrowth is not indicated.

How to Find Treatment for Your Candidiasis

If your Candida Spit Test indicates that you are suffering from a Candida overgrowth, it is important that you seek the care of a knowledgeable Chiropractic Physician. They can analyze the results of your test, find the cause of the Candida overgrowth, and recommend appropriate measures to control the Candida and return the balance between beneficial bacteria and Candida to your body.

Your Homework

Now that you understand how Candida overgrowth occurs and how your health can suffer from it, it is time to check the balance of your system.

Your homework for this chapter is to perform the Candida Spit Test. Record the results in the Workbook section of the book. If you see strings, cloudy specks, or your saliva floats to the bottom of the glass, it is time to seek appropriate care before Candidiasis destroys your health.

What's Next?

In the next chapter, you will learn how your posture affects your health and how to easily check it at home in front of a mirror.

Your good health is worth more than anything. You only have one body. Take care of it.

Chapter 13:

Postural Analysis – What Your Posture Tells You about Your Health

Chapter 13:

Postural Analysis – What Your Posture Tells You about Your Health

Posture is basically the positioning and alignment of your body with respect to gravity. Good posture is the proper positioning of your body that allows the forces of gravity to be distributed without putting too much stress on any one structure.

Your posture is a very important indicator of both the health of your spine and your organs. Even small changes in your posture can progress to severe problems. So, it is crucial that you learn how to recognize abnormalities in your posture early to be able to prevent them from worsening.

The Curves of Your Spine

Your Spine is made up of four natural curves: Your cervical (neck) curve, thoracic (upper back) curve, lumbar (low back) curve, and sacral/coccyx (tailbone) curve.

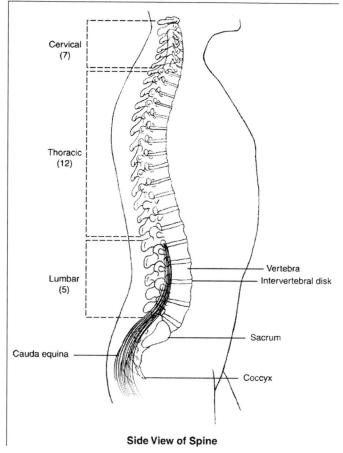

Side View of Spine

Your cervical and lumbar curves are called lordotic curves. This means that when you look at your spine form the side, they curve forward. Your thoracic and sacral curves are kyphotic, which means that when seen from the side, they curve backward.

The curves of the spine develop as a baby begins to lift their head and learns to crawl and walk. These curves are very important for both the health of your spine and your organs. They not only allow you to remain upright against gravity, they also acts as a spring for your spine. As you move, your curves bend and flex, allowing the stresses from the impact of walking, running, and other daily activities to be re-distributed. Without normal spinal curves, these stresses go directly into the spine, damaging bones, muscles, ligaments, and discs.

Your Curves and Your Posture

Normal curves lead to proper posture. At the same time, loss of these curves results in abnormal postural changes that result in increasing damage over time.

Your cervical, or neck, curve supports the heavy structure of your head over your body. In normal posture, this curve keeps your head back, with your ears centered over your shoulders. When you lose your cervical curve, your head moves forward on your shoulders. From the side, you will see that the hole for your ear will be located in front of your shoulders rather than directly over them. This is known as head forward posture.

Head forward posture has become more and more common, especially with the increasing number of people working at desks and on computers, where they look down all day. The problem with this is that head forward posture disrupts the alignment of your body, allowing the forces of gravity to put increased strain on your body. Every inch of head forward posture adds 10 pounds of extra strain to your neck. It's like carrying a bowling ball around on top of your head.

Your thoracic (upper back) curve is meant to hold you upright, keep your shoulders back, and open up the chest cavity so that your heart and lungs work optimally. If this curve changes and becomes exaggerated, or hyperkyphotic, your shoulders round, your back hunches over, and your chest cavity is compressed. This not only causes back pain but can lead to problems with your heart and lungs due to the constriction.

Your lumbar (low back) and sacral (tailbone) curves provide the foundation for your spine. They support the weight of your body whether you are standing or sitting. Any abnormalities in these curves can result in low back, hip, and leg pain as well as abdominal problems by causing compression and instability in the your lower spine.

Improper Posture – Causes and Symptoms

Postural changes usually happen slowly, over time. The small changes that happen on a daily basis result in muscle weakness and compensation, leading to larger postural abnormalities.

When you slouch, your body adapts to it and over days, months, and years it becomes a problem. Sitting at your desk for too long, watching TV on the couch, sitting in your car in traffic; all these result in muscles weakening, ligaments and tendons shortening, and the shape of your spine changing to compensate.

The longer postural abnormalities are left untreated, the worse they become. This is because when your posture changes, it affects all of the tissues attached to your spine. Some muscles, like your chest muscles, become shorter and tighter when your shoulders slump forward. Other muscles are stretched, irritated and weakened. As these structures change, they change the shape of your spine even more, compounding the problems.

You start to have pain, muscle tension, and headaches. You might ignore these problems at first. But, they don't go away. They only get worse. As postural abnormalities increase, you get less blood circulation to your extremities, more nerve compression, and decreased function of your organs, such as your heart and lungs.

Improper posture can cause instability and abnormal wear on your joints, leading to arthritis. It can even cause your spine to become fixed in an abnormal position, leading to scoliosis (an abnormal side curvature) of the spine and disc and nerve damage

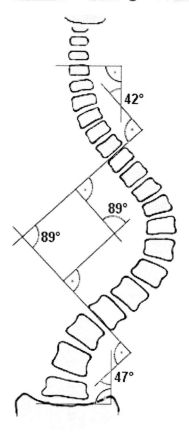

Spine Seen From the Back with Scoliosis (Side Curvature)

In children, instability of the spine is even more likely to result in scoliosis than in adults, so it is very important that a child's posture be regularly evaluated so potential future problems can be prevented.

What is Proper Posture?

With all the problems that result from bad posture, it is important to understand what good posture actually is. When we talk about proper posture, what we are looking for is the correct alignment of weight bearing joints. Generally posture is assessed from both the back and the side. Ideally, when looked at from behind, you spine should not have a lateral (side) curvature, your shoulders should be at the same height, as should your hips and fingertips, there should be no tilting of your head to one side, and your legs should look symmetrical without any angling of your knees or ankles.

From the side, your spine should show the smooth S-shape of the normal spinal curves. If an imaginary line was dropped from the top of your head, through the center of your body, it should pass through the tip of your shoulder, the center of your hip joint, slightly behind your knee joint, and through the center of your ankle.

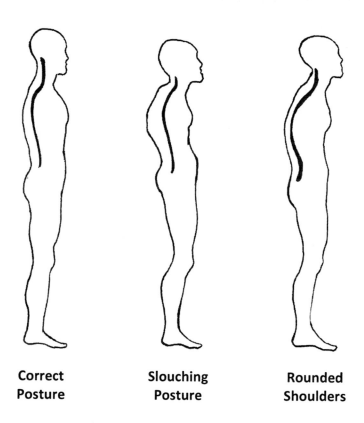

| Correct Posture | Slouching Posture | Rounded Shoulders |

In the picture above you can see the differences between a correct posture and some incorrect postures...

Here are some more images that show common issues with posture...

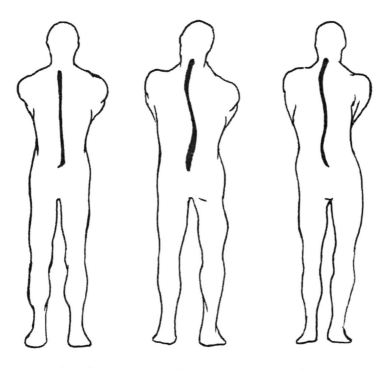

| Correct Posture | High Shoulder | High Hip |

And of course women can suffer the very same issues with posture as men...

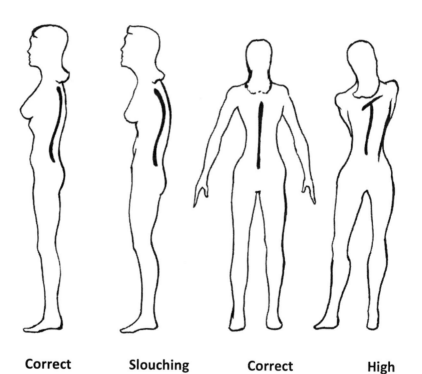

| Correct Posture | Slouching Posture | Correct Posture | High Shoulder |

When your body is in its proper alignment, your body weight is balanced over your spine and legs with minimum muscular effort. The pressures and stresses of daily activities are evenly distributed and there is no excess stress on your bones, muscles, discs, and ligaments. But, if your posture begins to deteriorate, more and more stress is placed on your body. Your muscles are strained, your ligaments are stretched, and the shape of your spine changes. Over time, these changes can become fixed as more problems develop.

When your spine is in proper alignment, your entire body works more optimally. Rounding of the shoulders occurs when your thoracic curve is exaggerated, causing muscle and back pain, headaches, and compressing the chest cavity. Alterations in the lumbar curve can also occur with a swayback posture where the lumbar curve is increased from its normal position. Excessive strain is put on the lower back, abdominal muscles weaken, and the risks of injury and instability are increased. You can also experience a flattening of the lumbar curve, causing tension in the low back, neck, and even the jaw.

Pregnancy can cause even more strain on the posture, so it's very important to be conscious of your posture throughout your pregnancy. The weight of the baby and your body's changing center of gravity can lead to your pelvis tilting forward, which causes strained abdominal muscles and excessive pressure on your bladder. The body changes of pregnancy can also lead to a rounding of your shoulders, which makes your breathing more difficult and causes indigestion.

It is vital during pregnancy to check your posture and work to maintain proper alignment. Your head should be up, with your ears over your shoulders and your chin lifted. Your abdominal muscles should be contracted to support the baby. And your buttocks should be tucked under, tilting your pubic bone slightly forward to maintain proper alignment.

When you look at your body in the mirror for proper alignment, you should see that the tips of your shoulders are even, that the fingertips of both arms are at the same level, and that your hip bones are level. Your ears should also be even, so that there is no tilting of your head to one side or the other.

If any of these areas is uneven, or one side higher than the other, this signifies that your body is out of proper alignment and excess strain is being put on your spine, muscles, ligaments, and organs.

The pictures on the next pages, showing your skeletal system, demonstrate the structures that you are looking for: the tips of your shoulders, or clavicles, the length of your fingertips, and the top of your pelvis, or hipbones.

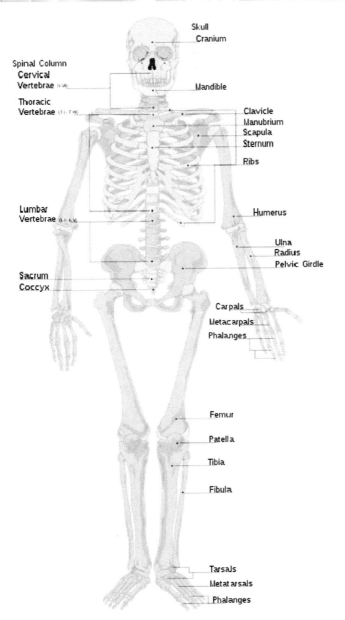

Skull
Cranium

Spinal Column
Cervical
Vertebrae (1-V8)

Mandible

Thoracic
Vertebrae (T1-T12)

Clavicle
Manubrium
Scapula
Sternum

Ribs

Lumbar
Vertebrae (L1-L5)

Humerus

Ulna
Radius
Pelvic Girdle

Sacrum
Coccyx

Carpals
Metacarpals
Phalanges

Femur

Patella

Tibia

Fibula

Tarsals
Metatarsals
Phalanges

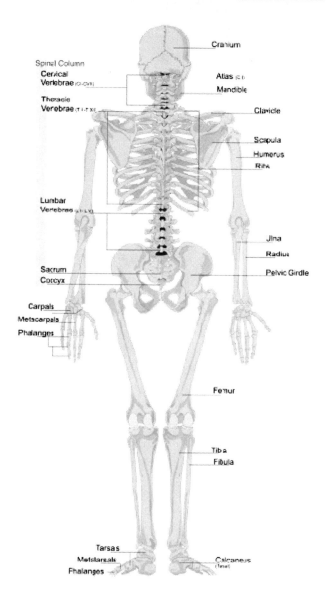

A healthy body, in proper alignment, has normal curves, even shoulders, ears, fingertips, and hips, and allows for easy of movement without pain or injury. Proper posture gives the spine stability and frees it to function properly.

Benefits of Proper Posture	
Decreased Muscle Tension	Decreased Pain
Increased Blood Flow	Improved Organ Function
Enhanced Balance	Improves Appearance
Engages Abdominal Muscles	Decreased Stress on Tissues

Postural Analysis – Step By Step Instruction

It is very easy to check your posture, your spouse's, or your child's posture at home. All you need is a mirror. If you are checking your own, you just have to observe yourself in the mirror. If you are checking someone else's posture, have them stand in front of the mirror with you behind them, where you can look over their shoulder.

1. Look in the mirror.
2. Check the height of your ears. Are they equal or is one higher than the other?

3. Check the height of your shoulders. You can place your fingertips on them to help.
    Are they equal or is one higher than the other?

4. Look at your hips. Place your thumbs, with your palms down, against the top of your hip bones. Is one higher than the other? Are they equal?

5. Let your arms drop to your sides. Note the height of your fingertips. Is one arm longer than the other or are they equal.

6. Record your observations in the Workbook section.

Tip: All areas should be at equal heights in proper posture. If you have any areas that are unequal (one higher than the other), this represents a postural abnormality.

How to Find Help for Improper Posture

Now that you understand how important your posture is not only to your spine but also to the health of your organs, you know why it is vital that you not ignore abnormalities in your posture. Small postural changes could be causing you pain, and decreased blood and nerve flow. They could also lead to even more severe problems including issues with your organ function.

If your postural analysis showed areas of improper posture, it is vital to seek the care of a qualified professional, knowledgeable in treating the posture, spine, muscles, and other tissues to find the cause of the problems and provide appropriate treatment to improve your posture and prevent worse issues from developing.

A Chiropractic Physician is trained to evaluate and treat all areas of the human body, with a special emphasis on treating the spine. Your Chiropractic Physician will be able to provide the best treatment possible to return your spine to optimum health and proper posture.

Your Homework

With all of the benefits that good posture offers your body, it is time to find out what clues your posture is offering about your health.

Your homework for this chapter is to perform the Postural Analysis. Record your findings in the Workbook section. And, if you find any postural abnormalities, you now know how to find the best care possible.

What's Next?

In the next chapter, you will learn about your feet, why they form your body's foundation, and how to easily check them with a simple test.

Good health is comprehensive and must encompass every portion of your being.

Chapter 14:

Flat Feet – How to Check Your Feet and Why It Is Important

Chapter 14:

Flat Feet – How to Check Your Feet and Why It Is Important

The term flat feet means that the arches of your feet are low or even absent. The medical term for this is "pes planus" or "pes valgus". The arch of your foot collapses and the entire sole of the foot comes into complete or near-complete contact with the ground. Having flat feet can lead to pain and problems not just in your feet but also in your ankles, knees, hips, and back.

In this chapter, you will learn more about the arches of your feet, what causes flat feet, and how to check your own feet at home to see if you suffer from this condition.

Your Feet and Arches

Your foot and ankle are complex structures that work together to form the foundation for your body. Just like the foundation of a house supports it, keeping it upright, your feet are the foundation that supports your body, allowing you to remain upright. Your foot and ankle are composed of more than 26 bones, 33 joints, and over a hundred muscles, tendons, and ligaments.

The arches of your foot are formed by your tarsal and metatarsal bones and held together by ligaments and tendons. These arches allow your foot to support your body weight and act as shock absorbers for your skeleton.

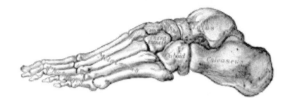

Your foot has two longitudinal arches and one transverse arch. Your arches are mobile, making walking and running easier. The medial longitudinal arch curves up, above the ground while the lateral longitudinal arch is much lower. The two longitudinal arches together support the transverse arch. Without these arches, your feet are unable to function normally, leading to problems throughout your skeletal system.

Having flat feet is normal in infants both because of the "baby fat" that covers the developing arch and the fact that the arch has not yet fully developed. Your arches develop in infancy and early childhood as normal muscle, bone, tendon, and ligament growth occur. Arches should form by the time a child is 2-3 years old.

Causes of Flat Feet

Flat feet are most often caused by excessive pronation. Pronation is when your foot's arch descends down and inward, or flattens, as your foot strikes the ground. Pronation is normal and necessary to your foot motion. But, excessive pronation leads to a loss of your foot's normal arches. Because of this, you lose the shock absorption that your arches provide, resulting in increased stress on your muscles, ligaments, and bones. This biomechanical imbalance can cause many painful foot conditions such as heel pain, plantar fasciitis, heel spurs, tendonitis, and even affect other parts of your body, including your knees, hips, and low back. It is estimated that 60-70% of the population suffers from excessive pronation due to flat feet.[32]

Flat feet can also result from loose ligaments. Ligaments are the bands of tissue that connect bones to each other. In your foot, your ligaments help to support your arches. Any condition that causes a loosening of the ligaments, such as pregnancy or rheumatoid arthritis, can result in loss of your feet's arches.

Another cause of flat feet is having one leg longer than the other (known as leg length inequality). When leg length inequality occurs, usually the foot on the longer leg will have a flatter arch, shortening the limb, to help balance the unevenness.

---

[32] Dr Foot. "1994" Flat feet. Retrieved May 17, 2012 from Dr Foot.co.uk http://www.drfoot.co.uk.htm

Preventive Care Through Home Testing

Injury, prolonged stress to the foot, obesity, and congenital foot abnormalities can all lead to fallen arches and flat feet.

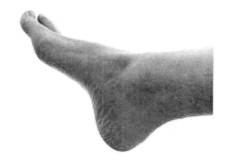

A foot with a normal arch

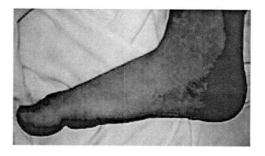

A flat foot

Runners especially suffer from flat feet due to both over-pronation during running as well as the repeated stress to the feet from running itself. Excessive pronation changes the proper alignment of the leg and can cause problems, including shin splints, back problems, and tendonitis of the knee.

Dr. Vladimir Gordin

How to Tell If You Have Flat Feet - Step By Step Instructions

The easiest way to tell if you have flat feet is by performing the Wet Footprint Test. It has been used for many years for home diagnosis. And, all you need to perform it is water and a smooth surface to stand on such as concrete or a thin piece of cardboard.

1. Wet the bottom of both of your feet.
2. Stand on a smooth, level surface, like concrete, thin cardboard, or heavy paper.
3. Check the imprint that your feet leave on the surface.
4. Record your results in the Workbook section of the book.
5. The larger the portion of the sole of the foot that leaves an imprint, the flatter your feet are.

If you see an imprint of your entire foot, you have flat feet. If the imprint does not show the middle of your foot, then you are not suffering from flat feet.

How to Find Help If You Have Flat Feet

If the results of your Wet Footprint Test reveal that you are suffering from flat feet, it is important to seek the care of a Chiropractic Physician for your condition.

Your Chiropractic Physician will be able to diagnose the cause of your flat feet, check your gait for over-pronation, look for loose ligaments and underlying conditions, and check for many more issues that can result in flat feet.

They will also be able to recommend an appropriate treatment plan to keep you from suffering from long-term problems such as knee, hip, and back injuries due to your flat feet.

Treatment may include orthotics, such as arch supports, muscle work, exercises, supplementation, and much more.

Your Chiropractic Physician will be able to set up a treatment plan that is specifically targeted to your individual needs.

Your Homework

Now you understand how flat feet can affect not only your feet but also your knees, hips, and back. And, you know how to easily discover whether or not you have flat feet that could be causing problems for your musculoskeletal system.

Your homework for this chapter is to perform the Wet Footprint Test and determine if the arches of your feet are normal or have dropped.

If the results of your test show that you have flat feet, you know the importance of getting treatment and how to find the right care.

What's Next?

In the next chapter, you will learn how breathing affects your health, the difference between chest breathing and diaphragmatic breathing, and how to check if you are breathing properly.

Remember, your health affects more than just the length of your life. It affects your family, your friends, and the quality of the life you live.

Chapter 15:

Proper Breathing – Your Breath and Your Health

Chapter 15:

Proper Breathing – Your Breath and Your Health

Your breathing can have a positive or negative effect on your health depending on whether or not you are breathing using your chest or your diaphragm. Your breathing method affects your oxygen intake, anxiety level, blood pressure, muscles, and much more.

Since your lung function can be used to predict your general health and how long you will live, it is very important to analyze how you breathe.[33]

Dr. Andrew Weil, MD, an internationally recognized expert on health says of the importance of proper breathing, "If I had to

---

[33] "Pulmonary Function is a Long Term Predictor of Mortality in General Population: 29 year Follow up of the Buffalo Health Study". [Pubmed]

limit my advice on healthier living to just one tip, it would be simply to learn how to breathe correctly."[34]

There are two types of breathing, diaphragmatic (stomach) and chest breathing.

Chest Breathing Causes

More than 50% of adults are chest breathers. And, more than 90% of sick people are chest breathers.[35] Few people in our society know how to breathe properly. Instead of breathing from our diaphragm, like we are supposed to, we are instead taught to suck in our stomach and puff out our chests to breathe.When you breathe from your chest rather than your diaphragm, you primarily use the middle and upper portion of your lungs, thereby not getting the health benefits of proper breathing.

Chest breathing can be triggered by anxiety, stress, fatigue, and lying down. Once chest breathing begins, it results in a cycle of hyperventilation that leads to more chest breathing. This is a dangerous feedback loop that can result in many medical problems.

---

[34] Stop Anxiety Attack Symptoms. "2012" Breathing – the proper technique. Retrieved May 18, 2012 from Stop Anxiety Attack Symptoms.com http://www.stop-anxiety-attack-symptoms.com/breathing.html

[35] Rakhimov, A. "2011" Chest (thoracic) breathing: effects, tests, and solutions. Retrieved from Normal Breathing.com http://www.normalbreathing.com/index-chest-breathing.php

Hyperventilation results in decreased oxygen delivery to your body's cells, tissues, and organs. Without the oxygen needed to function properly, your body's health deteriorates.

Chest Breathing Symptoms

When your body experiences hyperventilation, like in chest breathing, the first thing that happens, is that the blood vessels to your brain constrict. This reduces the oxygen available to your brain by approximately 50%. This can lead to mental fog, anxiety, panic attacks, agitation, and reduced motor skill control.[36]

Chest breathing can cause shortness of breath, chest pain from low heart oxygenation, sleep apnea, fatigue, constipation, and a stuffy nose. Since chest breathing recruits muscles that otherwise would be relaxed, it can result in tension, pain, and headache. Chest breathing also makes exhaling completely difficult, leaving you feeling short of breath. Compared to proper, diaphragmatic breathing, chest breathing is very inefficient, making breathing feel more difficult and you feel more tired.

---

[36] Peters, D. "2012" Upper chest breathing. Retrieved May 19, 2012 from Murphy's Law Neuromuscular Therapy
http://www.murphyslawmassagetherapy.com/upper-chest-breathing

Physical Signs of Chest Breathing

Jaw or Facial Tension

Postural Tension

Raised Shoulders

Protracted Scapula (Shoulder Blades)

Kyphosis (Hunched Back)

Scoliosis

Chest breathing ultimately limits the ability of your rib cage to expand, hampering your ability to breathe at all. Since you are unable to completely exhale, stale air remains trapped in your lungs, less oxygen reaches your cells, tissues, and organs, leading to diseases of your heart and lungs.

Benefits of Diaphragmatic Breathing

Diaphragmatic breathing, sometimes called stomach or abdominal breathing is the proper way to breathe and has many health benefits. In diaphragmatic breathing, your diaphragm contracts, expanding your stomach and forcing air into your lungs. The best examples of diaphragmatic breathing are babies. When babies breathe, their stomachs move up and down as they use their diaphragm, not their chest.

This type of breathing uses the lower, middle, and upper lobes of the lungs unlike chest breathing, which only engages the lower and middle lobes. Bringing air into the lower portion of the lungs, where oxygen exchange is most efficient helps to slow the heart rate, decrease blood pressure, relax muscles, and calm anxiety.[37] The upper 10% of your lungs are able to transport less than 6 ml of oxygen per minute while the lower 10% of your lungs are capable of transporting more than 40 ml of oxygen per minute. This means that the lower lobes of your lungs are approximately 6-7 times more effective in transporting oxygen and oxygenating your blood.

Studies have even linked focused, diaphragmatic breathing with reduced hot flashes in menopausal women, reduced symptoms of PMS, and improvement in the symptoms of chronic pain.

Diaphragmatic breathing reduces tight chest muscles which relieves muscle tension, chest pain, and anxiety. It opens up the chest, allowing for deeper breathing, reducing respiratory problems like asthma and bronchitis.

Your heart, brain, and other organs also benefit from diaphragmatic breathing, since it increases the oxygenation of your blood, allowing your organs to receive the oxygen they need to function properly.

Diaphragmatic breathing even helps your body with lymphatic drainage, eliminating toxins, and improving your immune

---

[37] Krucoff, C. "Better living through belly breathing". The Seattle Times. May 10, 2000. Section C3.

system. It also helps your urinary system by allowing fluids to be eliminated through your breathing, reducing edema and stress on your kidneys.

How Do You Breathe? – Step By Step Instructions to Test Your Breathing Type

Considering how detrimental chest breathing is to your health whereas diaphragmatic breathing offers so many health benefits, it is important to learn what your breathing type is. It is a very simple test that you can do at home in front of a mirror and requires no equipment. The test can be done both standing up, in front of a mirror, or lying down.

Standing Test

1. Stand in front of a mirror.
2. Relax completely so that your breathing won't fluctuate.
3. Put your right hand on your stomach and your left hand on your chest.
4. Breathe normally.
5. Observe your breathing for 20-30 seconds with both hands in place.
6. If your right hand rises more, you are a stomach breather.
7. If your left hand rises more, you are a chest breather.

8. Record your results in the Workbook section of the book.

Test Lying Down

1. Lie on your back, face up.
2. Place one hand on your chest and the other on your stomach.
3. Watch your hands as you breathe.

The sequence of movements for your hands in normal breathing is stomach up, chest up on the inhale and chest down then stomach down on the exhale.

Finding Help to Change Your Chest Breathing

If after performing the breathing test, you discover that you are a chest breather, it is time to seek care from a Chiropractic Physician experienced in treating this problem. A multi-disciplinary practice is a good choice since you will find a Chiropractic Physician who can analyze your breathing patterns, discover the underlying causes, teach you proper breathing techniques, and set up a treatment plan to prevent chest breathing from damaging your health.

Your Homework

In this chapter, you learned the difference between chest breathing and diaphragmatic breathing. You also discovered why proper, diaphragmatic breathing is crucial to living a healthy life.

Your homework for this chapter is to perform the breathing test to determine whether you are a chest breather or a diaphragmatic breather. Record your results in the Workbook section of the book. If your results indicate that you are a chest breather, you now know how to find the care you need to prevent chest breathing from damaging your cells, organs, tissues, and your life.

What's Next?

You have finished the last test in this book and taken another step toward a healthier life. In the next section, we will briefly discuss what we have learned and when to seek care for any health problems. When you perform your health checks, don't forget to include your family and children. A lifetime of good health starts early. In the next chapter, we will briefly review when and how to seek the best care possible if any of your tests have not shown optimal results.

Congratulate yourself. You have taken a giant step toward a healthier life.

Conclusion

You have now learned 14 different tests to help you easily monitor your health at home. By performing these tests and keeping track of your results, you can discover issues in your health early and get treatment before they become serious and symptomatic. By performing these tests, you have taken back control of your health and well-being and made a commitment to living a healthier life.

If any of the tests you have dove have shown abnormal results, it is important that you seek appropriate care to prevent the problems from progressing. A Chiropractic Physician, experienced in treating the body as a whole is a good choice. They are able to analyze all aspects of your health, including your spine, muscles, diet, exercise, supplements, hormones, organ function, stress, fatigue, depression, and more. By taking this holistic approach, your Chiropractic Physician can discover and treat the underlying cause of your health issues, not just the symptoms.

Now that you have learned so much about your health, you will be more aware of how your body works and the difference between optimal and sub-optimal health.

Preventive Care Through Home Testing

If your health changes or you experience any health issues outside of the tests you have learned in this book, it is vital to seek qualified, professional care as soon as possible. By being proactive with your health rather than reactive, you can live a much healthier life.

In the next section, you will find a Symptom Survey Form. It contains 224 symptoms that a healthy person should not have. Complete the form and, if you are experiencing any of the symptoms, seek out an experienced professional trained in the use of the form to interpret the results and provide appropriate care.

Appendix B contains the Workbook section of the book, which you have been using to record the results of your home testing. Should you need to see a Physician, be sure to take your Workbook with you to allow them to fully analyze your results.

If your test results are in the normal range, continue to perform the tests on a regular basis to monitor for any changes.

Congratulations! By completing the tests in this book, you have committed to living a healthier life.

Appendix A

Symptom Survey Form

The following pages contain a Symptom Survey Form for you to fill out. It lists 224 symptoms which a healthy person should not have. If after completing the survey, you find that you are experiencing any of the symptoms listed, you should seek out a qualified professional trained in the use of this form to interpret your results and provide appropriate recommendations and treatment.

To complete the survey, read each symptom. If you have experienced the symptom, circle the number that corresponds to the level of your symptoms.

Circle 1 if you have mild symptoms that occur only once or twice a year.

Circle 2 if you have moderate symptoms that occur several times a month.

Circle 3 if you have severe symptoms that you are aware of almost constantly.

Circle nothing if you do not experience the symptom.

Preventive Care Through Home Testing

On the last page, list your 5 main physical complaints in the order of their importance.

If you need to seek care, make sure to take this form with you so that a qualified healthcare professional can fully evaluate your health.

Symptom Survey Form:

GROUP ONE

1 - **1 2 3** Acid foods upset

2 - **1 2 3** Get chilled, often

3 - **1 2 3** "Lump" in throat

4 - **1 2 3** Dry mouth-eyes-nose

5 - **1 2 3** Pulse speeds after meal

6 - **1 2 3** Keyed up – fail to calm

7 - **1 2 3** Cuts heal slowly

8 - **1 2 3** Gag easily

9 - **1 2 3** Unable to relax; startles easily

10 - **1 2 3** Extremities cold, clammy

11 - **1 2 3** Strong light irritates

12 - **1 2 3** Urine amount reduced

13 - **1 2 3** Heart pounds after retiring

14 - **1 2 3** "Nervous" stomach

15 - **1 2 3** Appetite reduced

16 - **1 2 3** Cold sweats often

17 - **1 2 3** Fever easily raised

18 - **1 2 3** Neuralgia-like pains

19 - **1 2 3** Staring, blinks little

20 - **1 2 3** Sour stomach frequent

(continued on the next page)

GROUP TWO

21 - **1 2 3** Joint stiffness after arising

22 - **1 2 3** Muscle-leg-toe cramps at night

23 - **1 2 3** "Butterfly" stomach, cramps

24 - **1 2 3** Eyes or nose watery

25 - **1 2 3** Eyes blink often

26 - **1 2 3** Eyelids swollen, puffy

27 - **1 2 3** Indigestion soon after meals

28 - **1 2 3** Always seems hungry; feels "lightheaded" often

29 - **1 2 3** Digestion rapid

30 - **1 2 3** Vomiting frequent

31 - **1 2 3** Hoarseness frequent

32 - **1 2 3** Breathing irregular

33 - **1 2 3** Pulse slow; feels "irregular"

34 - **1 2 3** Gagging reflex slow

35 - **1 2 3** Difficulty swallowing

36 - **1 2 3** Constipation, diarrhea alternating

37 - **1 2 3** "Slow starter"

38 - **1 2 3** Get "chilled" infrequently

39 - **1 2 3** Perspire easily

40 - **1 2 3** Circulation poor, sensitive to cold

41 - **1 2 3** Subject to colds, asthma, bronchitis

(continued on the next page)

GROUP THREE

42 - **1 2 3** Eat when nervous

43 - **1 2 3** Excessive appetite

44 - **1 2 3** Hungry between meals

45 - **1 2 3** Irritable before meals

46 - **1 2 3** Get "shaky" if hungry

47 - **1 2 3** Fatigue, eating relieves

48 - **1 2 3** "Lightheaded" if meals delayed

49 - **1 2 3** Heart palpitates if meals missed or delayed

50 - **1 2 3** Afternoon headaches

51 - **1 2 3** Overeating sweets upsets

52 - **1 2 3** Awaken after few hours sleep – hard to get back to sleep

53 - **1 2 3** Crave candy or coffee in afternoons

54 - **1 2 3** Moods of depression – "blues" or melancholy

55 - **1 2 3** Abnormal craving for sweets or snacks

(continued on the next page)

GROUP FOUR

56 - **1 2 3** Hands and feet go to sleep easily, numbness

57 - **1 2 3** Sigh frequently, "air hunger"

58 - **1 2 3** Aware of "breathing heavily"

59 - **1 2 3** High altitude discomfort

60 - **1 2 3** Opens windows in closed room

61 - **1 2 3** Susceptible to colds and fevers

62 - **1 2 3** Afternoon "yawner"

63 - **1 2 3** Get "drowsy" often

64 - **1 2 3** Swollen ankles worse at night

65 - **1 2 3** Muscle cramps, worse during exercise; get "charley horses"

66 - **1 2 3** Shortness of breath on exertion

67 - **1 2 3** Dull pain in chest or radiating into left arm, worse on exertion.

68 - **1 2 3** Bruise easily, "black and blue" spots

69 - **1 2 3** Tendency to anemia

70 - **1 2 3** "Nose bleeds" frequent

71 - **1 2 3** Noises in head, or "ringing in ears"

72 - **1 2 3** Tension under the breastbone, or feeling of "tightness" worse on exertion

(continued on the next page)

GROUP FIVE

73 - **1 2 3** Dizziness

74 - **1 2 3** Dry Skin

75 - **1 2 3** Burning feet

76 - **1 2 3** Blurred vision

77 - **1 2 3** Itching skin and feet

78 - **1 2 3** Excessive falling hair

79 - **1 2 3** Frequent skin rashes

80 - **1 2 3** Bitter, metallic taste in mouth in mornings

81 - **1 2 3** Bowel movements painful or difficult

82 - **1 2 3** Worrier, feels insecure

83 - **1 2 3** Feeling queasy; headache over eyes

84 - **1 2 3** Greasy foods upset

85 - **1 2 3** Stools light-colored

86 - **1 2 3** Skin peels on foot soles

87 - **1 2 3** Pain between shoulder blades

88 - **1 2 3** Use laxatives

89 - **1 2 3** Stools alternate from soft to watery

90 - **1 2 3** History of gallbladder attacks or gallstones

91 - **1 2 3** Sneezing attacks

92 - **1 2 3** Dreaming, nightmare type bad dreams

93 - **1 2 3** Bad breath (halitosis)

94 - **1 2 3** Milk products cause distress

95 - **1 2 3** Sensitive to hot weather

96 - **1 2 3** Burning or itching anus

97 - **1 2 3** Crave sweets

(continued on the next page)

GROUP SIX

98 - **1 2 3** Loss of taste for meat

99 - **1 2 3** Lower bowel gas several hours after eating

100 - **1 2 3** Burning stomach sensations, eating relieves

101 - **1 2 3** Coated tongue

102 - **1 2 3** Pass large amounts of foul smelling gas

103 - **1 2 3** Indigestion ½ - 1 hour after eating; may be up to 3 – 4 hrs.

104 - **1 2 3** Mucous colitis or "irritable bowel"

105 - **1 2 3** Gas shortly after eating

106 - **1 2 3** Stomach "bloating" after eating

GROUP SEVEN   (A)

107 - **1 2 3** Insomnia

108 - **1 2 3** Nervousness

109 - **1 2 3** Can't gain weight

110 - **1 2 3** Intolerance to heat

111 - **1 2 3** Highly emotional

112 - **1 2 3** Flush easily

113 - **1 2 3** Night sweats

114 - **1 2 3** Thin, moist skin

115 - **1 2 3** Inward trembling

116 - **1 2 3** Heart palpitates

117 - **1 2 3** Increased appetite without weight gain

118 - **1 2 3** Pulse fast at rest

119 - **1 2 3** Eyelids and face twitch

120 - **1 2 3** Irritable and restless

121 - **1 2 3** Can't work under pressure

(continued on the next page)

GROUP SEVEN (B)

122 - **1 2 3** Increase in weight

123 - **1 2 3** Decrease in appetite

124 - **1 2 3** Fatigue easily

125 - **1 2 3** Ringing in ears

126 - **1 2 3** Sleepy during day

127 - **1 2 3** Sensitive to cold

128 - **1 2 3** Dry or scaly skin

129 - **1 2 3** Constipation

130 - **1 2 3** Mental sluggishness

131 - **1 2 3** Hair coarse, falls out

132 - **1 2 3** Headaches upon arising wear off during day

133 - **1 2 3** Slow pulse, below 65

134 - **1 2 3** Frequency of urination

135 - **1 2 3** Impaired hearing

136 - **1 2 3** Reduced initiative

GROUP SEVEN (C)

137 - **1 2 3** Failing memory

138 - **1 2 3** Low blood pressure

139 - **1 2 3** Increased sex drive

140 - **1 2 3** Headaches, "splitting or rending" type

141 - **1 2 3** Decreased sugar tolerance

GROUP SEVEN (D)

142 - **1 2 3** Abnormal thirst

143 - **1 2 3** Bloating of abdomen

144 - **1 2 3** Weight gain around hips or waist

145 - **1 2 3** Sex drive reduced or lacking

146 - **1 2 3** Tendency to ulcers, colitis

147 - **1 2 3** Increased sugar tolerance

148 - **1 2 3** Women: menstrual disorders

149 - **1 2 3** Young girls: lack of menstrual function

GROUP SEVEN   (E)

150 - **1 2 3** Dizziness

151 - **1 2 3** Headaches

152 - **1 2 3** Hot flashes

153 - **1 2 3** Increased blood pressure

154 - **1 2 3** Hair growth on face or body (female)

155 - **1 2 3** Sugar in urine (not diabetes)

156 - **1 2 3** Masculine tendencies (female)

GROUP SEVEN   (F)

157 - **1 2 3** Weakness, dizziness

158 - **1 2 3** Chronic fatigue

159 - **1 2 3** Low blood pressure

160 - **1 2 3** Nails weak, ridged

161 - **1 2 3** Tendency to hives

162 - **1 2 3** Arthritic tendencies

163 - **1 2 3** Perspiration increase

164 - **1 2 3** Bowel disorders

165 - **1 2 3** Poor circulation

166 - **1 2 3** Swollen ankles

167 - **1 2 3** Crave salt

168 - **1 2 3** Brown spots or bronzing of skin

169 - **1 2 3** Allergies – tendency to asthma

170 - **1 2 3** Weakness after colds, influenza

171 - **1 2 3** Exhaustion – muscular and nervous

172 - **1 2 3** Respiratory disorders

(continued on the next page)

FEMALE ONLY

200 - **1 2 3** Very easily fatigued

201 - **1 2 3** Premenstrual tension

202 - **1 2 3** Painful menses

203 - **1 2 3** Depressed feelings

204 - **1 2 3** Menstruation excessive and prolonged

205 - **1 2 3** Painful breasts

206 - **1 2 3** Menstruate too frequently

207 - **1 2 3** Vaginal discharge

208 - **1 2 3** Hysterectomy/ovaries removed

209 - **1 2 3** Menopausal hot flashes

210 - **1 2 3** Menses scanty or missed

211 - **1 2 3** Acne, worse at menses

212 - **1 2 3** Depression of long standing

MALE ONLY

213 - **1 2 3** Prostate trouble

214 - **1 2 3** Urination difficult or dribbling

215 - **1 2 3** Night urination frequent

216 - **1 2 3** Depression

217 - **1 2 3** Pain on inside of legs or heels

218 - **1 2 3** Feeling of incomplete bowel evacuation

219 - **1 2 3** Lack of energy

220 - **1 2 3** Migrating aches and pains

221 - **1 2 3** Tire too easily

222 - **1 2 3** Avoids activity

223 - **1 2 3** Leg nervousness at night

224 - **1 2 3** Diminished sex drive

(continued on the next page)

IMPORTANT

Please list below the five main physical complaints you
have in order of their importance:

1. _____

2. _____

3. _____

4. _____

5. _____

Appendix B

Workbook

Chapter 2 – Blood Pressure

Record the blood pressure readings for both your right and left arm for 14 days. Circle any abnormal readings, both high and low. Also circle any difference in readings between sides of more than 10mm.

Date	BP Right Arm	BP Left Arm	Difference> 10mm Yes/No

Continued on the Next Page...

Date	BP Right Arm	BP Left Arm	Difference> 10mm Yes/No

Chapter 3 – Pulse Oximetry

Measure your pulse ox every day for at least 14 days and record. Circle any readings that are below 99%.

Date						
Pulse Ox %						

Date						
Pulse Ox %						

Date						
Pulse Ox %						

Chapter 4 – Allergy Pulse Diagnostic Test

Measure your pulse before you get out of bed and again right before you eat. Eat only one type of food at a time. Measure your pulse 30 and 60 minutes after eating. Repeat with a different food.

An increase in pulse rate of more than 10 beats per minute indicates a possible food allergy.

Day 1:

Food Type	Pulse in AM	Pulse Prior to Eating	Pulse 30 minutes after eating	Pulse 60 minutes after eating	Change in Pulse Rate

Day 2:

Food Type	Pulse in AM	Pulse Prior to Eating	Pulse 30 minutes after eating	Pulse 60 minutes after eating	Change in Pulse Rate

Day 3:

Food Type	Pulse in AM	Pulse Prior to Eating	Pulse 30 minutes after eating	Pulse 60 minutes after eating	Change in Pulse Rate

Chapter 5 – Ragland's Test

Take your blood pressure in the appropriate positions, using an automatic blood pressure cuff. Record your results and note the differences in pressure between position.

If you systolic does not rise from sitting to standing by 4-12 mm, it indicates adrenal fatigue. If your systolic does not drop from sitting to lying down by 4-12 mm, it indicates a problem with your kidneys.

Date	Blood Pressure Sitting (1)	Blood Pressure Standing (2)	Blood Pressure Lying Down (3)	Difference between sitting and standing (2 minus 1)	Difference between sitting and lying down (1 minus 3)

Chapter 6 - Pin Light Pupillary Test

Look in a mirror as you shine a penlight or flashlight in from the side of your eye for 30 seconds. Check both eyes. Check the box that appropriately describes the reaction of each eye. If your pupil remains constricted, adrenal fatigue is not indicated. If your pupil constricts but then dilates, or enlarges, again or "pulses" between constriction and dilation, you could be suffering from adrenal fatigue.

Reaction	Right Eye	Left Eye
Pupil Remains Constricted		
Pupil Constricts but then Dilates Again		
Pupil "Pulses" between Constriction and Dilation		

Chapter 7 – Calcium Blood Pressure Cuff Test

In this test, you use a blood pressure cuff around your calf to determine if the calcium level in your muscles is low. If you have no cramping as you pump up the cuff to 220 mm, your calcium levels are normal. If you have cramping between 180-220 mm, your calcium level is borderline low. Cramping below 180 mm indicates calcium deficiency.

Note: Any difference in cramping between legs can indicate a vascular problem.

Date:	Right Leg	Left Leg
Cramping Yes/No		
Reading on Blood Pressure Cuff at Time of Cramping		

Chapter 8 – Broda Barnes Body Temperature Test

For men and for women who no longer have menstrual cycles, chart your morning body temperature for 10 days.

Women with menstrual cycles, chart for a full 30 days of your cycle.

For your convenience, start on Day 1. The charts are on the following pages...

PLEASE NOTE: If test results are near the edges of the chart for more than one or two days, medical attention should be sought.

If readings are "off the chart" then *immediate* attention is warranted.

Preventive Care Through Home Testing

This chart has the temperature measurements in Fahrenheit.

Day	1	2	3	4	5	6	7	8	9	10	11	12	13	14	15
	99	99	99	99	99	99	99	99	99	99	99	99	99	99	99
	9	9	9	9	9	9	9	9	9	9	9	9	9	9	9
	8	8	8	8	8	8	8	8	8	8	8	8	8	8	8
	7	7	7	7	7	7	7	7	7	7	7	7	7	7	7
	6	6	6	6	6	6	6	6	6	6	6	6	6	6	6
	5	5	5	5	5	5	5	5	5	5	5	5	5	5	5
	4	4	4	4	4	4	4	4	4	4	4	4	4	4	4
	3	3	3	3	3	3	3	3	3	3	3	3	3	3	3
	2	2	2	2	2	2	2	2	2	2	2	2	2	2	2
	1	1	1	1	1	1	1	1	1	1	1	1	1	1	1
	98	98	98	98	98	98	98	98	98	98	98	98	98	98	98
	9	9	9	9	9	9	9	9	9	9	9	9	9	9	9
	8	8	8	8	8	8	8	8	8	8	8	8	8	8	8
	7	7	7	7	7	7	7	7	7	7	7	7	7	7	7
	6	6	6	6	6	6	6	6	6	6	6	6	6	6	6
	5	5	5	5	5	5	5	5	5	5	5	5	5	5	5
	4	4	4	4	4	4	4	4	4	4	4	4	4	4	4
	3	3	3	3	3	3	3	3	3	3	3	3	3	3	3
	2	2	2	2	2	2	2	2	2	2	2	2	2	2	2
	1	1	1	1	1	1	1	1	1	1	1	1	1	1	1
	97	97	97	97	97	97	97	97	97	97	97	97	97	97	97
	9	9	9	9	9	9	9	9	9	9	9	9	9	9	9
	8	8	8	8	8	8	8	8	8	8	8	8	8	8	8
	7	7	7	7	7	7	7	7	7	7	7	7	7	7	7
	6	6	6	6	6	6	6	6	6	6	6	6	6	6	6
	5	5	5	5	5	5	5	5	5	5	5	5	5	5	5
	4	4	4	4	4	4	4	4	4	4	4	4	4	4	4
	3	3	3	3	3	3	3	3	3	3	3	3	3	3	3
	2	2	2	2	2	2	2	2	2	2	2	2	2	2	2
	1	1	1	1	1	1	1	1	1	1	1	1	1	1	1
	96	96	96	96	96	96	96	96	96	96	96	96	96	96	96
Day	1	2	3	4	5	6	7	8	9	10	11	12	13	14	15

Dr. Vladimir Gordin

Day	16	17	18	19	20	21	22	23	24	25	26	27	28	29	30
	99	99	99	99	99	99	99	99	99	99	99	99	99	99	99
	9	9	9	9	9	9	9	9	9	9	9	9	9	9	9
	8	8	8	8	8	8	8	8	8	8	8	8	8	8	8
	7	7	7	7	7	7	7	7	7	7	7	7	7	7	7
	6	6	6	6	6	6	6	6	6	6	6	6	6	6	6
	5	5	5	5	5	5	5	5	5	5	5	5	5	5	5
	4	4	4	4	4	4	4	4	4	4	4	4	4	4	4
	3	3	3	3	3	3	3	3	3	3	3	3	3	3	3
	2	2	2	2	2	2	2	2	2	2	2	2	2	2	2
	1	1	1	1	1	1	1	1	1	1	1	1	1	1	1
	98	98	98	98	98	98	98	98	98	98	98	98	98	98	98
	9	9	9	9	9	9	9	9	9	9	9	9	9	9	9
	8	8	8	8	8	8	8	8	8	8	8	8	8	8	8
	7	7	7	7	7	7	7	7	7	7	7	7	7	7	7
	6	6	6	6	6	6	6	6	6	6	6	6	6	6	6
	5	5	5	5	5	5	5	5	5	5	5	5	5	5	5
	4	4	4	4	4	4	4	4	4	4	4	4	4	4	4
	3	3	3	3	3	3	3	3	3	3	3	3	3	3	3
	2	2	2	2	2	2	2	2	2	2	2	2	2	2	2
	1	1	1	1	1	1	1	1	1	1	1	1	1	1	1
	97	97	97	97	97	97	97	97	97	97	97	97	97	97	97
	9	9	9	9	9	9	9	9	9	9	9	9	9	9	9
	8	8	8	8	8	8	8	8	8	8	8	8	8	8	8
	7	7	7	7	7	7	7	7	7	7	7	7	7	7	7
	6	6	6	6	6	6	6	6	6	6	6	6	6	6	6
	5	5	5	5	5	5	5	5	5	5	5	5	5	5	5
	4	4	4	4	4	4	4	4	4	4	4	4	4	4	4
	3	3	3	3	3	3	3	3	3	3	3	3	3	3	3
	2	2	2	2	2	2	2	2	2	2	2	2	2	2	2
	1	1	1	1	1	1	1	1	1	1	1	1	1	1	1
	96	96	96	96	96	96	96	96	96	96	96	96	96	96	96
Day	16	17	18	19	20	21	22	23	24	25	26	27	28	29	30

This chart has the temperature measurements in Celsius.

Day	1	2	3	4	5	6	7	8	9	10	11	12	13	14	15
	37	37	37	37	37	37	37	37	37	37	37	37	37	37	37
	9	9	9	9	9	9	9	9	9	9	9	9	9	9	9
	8	8	8	8	8	8	8	8	8	8	8	8	8	8	8
	7	7	7	7	7	7	7	7	7	7	7	7	7	7	7
	6	6	6	6	6	6	6	6	6	6	6	6	6	6	6
	5	5	5	5	5	5	5	5	5	5	5	5	5	5	5
	4	4	4	4	4	4	4	4	4	4	4	4	4	4	4
	3	3	3	3	3	3	3	3	3	3	3	3	3	3	3
	2	2	2	2	2	2	2	2	2	2	2	2	2	2	2
	1	1	1	1	1	1	1	1	1	1	1	1	1	1	1
	36	36	36	36	36	36	36	36	36	36	36	36	36	36	36
	9	9	9	9	9	9	9	9	9	9	9	9	9	9	9
	8	8	8	8	8	8	8	8	8	8	8	8	8	8	8
	7	7	7	7	7	7	7	7	7	7	7	7	7	7	7
	6	6	6	6	6	6	6	6	6	6	6	6	6	6	6
	5	5	5	5	5	5	5	5	5	5	5	5	5	5	5
	4	4	4	4	4	4	4	4	4	4	4	4	4	4	4
	3	3	3	3	3	3	3	3	3	3	3	3	3	3	3
	2	2	2	2	2	2	2	2	2	2	2	2	2	2	2
	1	1	1	1	1	1	1	1	1	1	1	1	1	1	1
	35	35	35	35	35	35	35	35	35	35	35	35	35	35	35
	9	9	9	9	9	9	9	9	9	9	9	9	9	9	9
	8	8	8	8	8	8	8	8	8	8	8	8	8	8	8
	7	7	7	7	7	7	7	7	7	7	7	7	7	7	7
	6	6	6	6	6	6	6	6	6	6	6	6	6	6	6
	5	5	5	5	5	5	5	5	5	5	5	5	5	5	5
	4	4	4	4	4	4	4	4	4	4	4	4	4	4	4
	3	3	3	3	3	3	3	3	3	3	3	3	3	3	3
	2	2	2	2	2	2	2	2	2	2	2	2	2	2	2
	1	1	1	1	1	1	1	1	1	1	1	1	1	1	1
	34	34	34	34	34	34	34	34	34	34	34	34	34	34	34
Day	1	2	3	4	5	6	7	8	9	10	11	12	13	14	15

Day	16	17	18	19	20	21	22	23	24	25	26	27	28	29	30
	37	37	37	37	37	37	37	37	37	37	37	37	37	37	37
	9	9	9	9	9	9	9	9	9	9	9	9	9	9	9
	8	8	8	8	8	8	8	8	8	8	8	8	8	8	8
	7	7	7	7	7	7	7	7	7	7	7	7	7	7	7
	6	6	6	6	6	6	6	6	6	6	6	6	6	6	6
	5	5	5	5	5	5	5	5	5	5	5	5	5	5	5
	4	4	4	4	4	4	4	4	4	4	4	4	4	4	4
	3	3	3	3	3	3	3	3	3	3	3	3	3	3	3
	2	2	2	2	2	2	2	2	2	2	2	2	2	2	2
	1	1	1	1	1	1	1	1	1	1	1	1	1	1	1
	36	36	36	36	36	36	36	36	36	36	36	36	36	36	36
	9	9	9	9	9	9	9	9	9	9	9	9	9	9	9
	8	8	8	8	8	8	8	8	8	8	8	8	8	8	8
	7	7	7	7	7	7	7	7	7	7	7	7	7	7	7
	6	6	6	6	6	6	6	6	6	6	6	6	6	6	6
	5	5	5	5	5	5	5	5	5	5	5	5	5	5	5
	4	4	4	4	4	4	4	4	4	4	4	4	4	4	4
	3	3	3	3	3	3	3	3	3	3	3	3	3	3	3
	2	2	2	2	2	2	2	2	2	2	2	2	2	2	2
	1	1	1	1	1	1	1	1	1	1	1	1	1	1	1
	35	35	35	35	35	35	35	35	35	35	35	35	35	35	35
	9	9	9	9	9	9	9	9	9	9	9	9	9	9	9
	8	8	8	8	8	8	8	8	8	8	8	8	8	8	8
	7	7	7	7	7	7	7	7	7	7	7	7	7	7	7
	6	6	6	6	6	6	6	6	6	6	6	6	6	6	6
	5	5	5	5	5	5	5	5	5	5	5	5	5	5	5
	4	4	4	4	4	4	4	4	4	4	4	4	4	4	4
	3	3	3	3	3	3	3	3	3	3	3	3	3	3	3
	2	2	2	2	2	2	2	2	2	2	2	2	2	2	2
	1	1	1	1	1	1	1	1	1	1	1	1	1	1	1
	34	34	34	34	34	34	34	34	34	34	34	34	34	34	34
Day	16	17	18	19	20	21	22	23	24	25	26	27	28	29	30

Preventive Care Through Home Testing
Chapter 9 – Iodine Skin Test

After painting a 2 inch patch of iodine on your inner thigh or upper arm, monitor how long the patch remains on your skin. Record the date and check the appropriate box for the length of time the patch remained.

If the patch was still there after 24 hours, you are not iodine deficient.

If the patch disappeared prior to the 12 hour time period, your iodine is low.

If the patch disappeared prior to the 8 hour time period, you are very iodine deficient.

Date/ Time Lasted						
>24 hours						
<12 hours						
<8 hours						

Chapter 10 – Zinc Nail Test

After looking at your nails for white spots, bands, or lines, record your observations here. You can also take a picture of your nails are draw what you see in the place provided on the next page.

Observations:

_____

_____

_____

_____

_____

_____

_____

Draw pictures or write descriptions here. Be sure to number each nail.

Chapter 11 – Zinc Oral Solution Test

After holding the zinc oral solution in your mouth for 10 seconds, rate your perception on the following scale.

1. No specific taste, tastes like water – indicates major zinc deficiency.
2. You don't notice a taste immediately but within 10 seconds, you notice a dry or metallic taste – indicates moderate zinc deficiency.
3. You notice an immediate, strong taste that is not necessarily unpleasant but builds over the 10 second time period – indicates minor zinc deficiency.
4. You notice an immediate, strong, unpleasant taste – indicates no zinc deficiency.

Check the box for the rating that most closely indicates your perception and record the date of the test.

Date/ Perception Grade				
1				
2				
3				
4				

Chapter 12 – Candida Spit Test

Follow the instructions in the chapter to perform the Candida Spit Test. Make sure to do the test as soon as you wake up. Circle any abnormal findings as seen on the illustration below (legs, cloudy specks, saliva floating to the bottom). If you have no abnormal findings, write "Negative".

SALIVA TEST

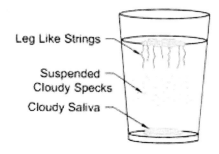

Leg Like Strings

Suspended Cloudy Specks

Cloudy Saliva

Date: _____

Findings: _____

SALIVA TEST

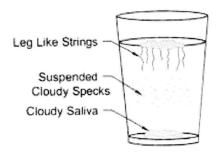

Leg Like Strings

Suspended
Cloudy Specks

Cloudy Saliva

Date: _____

Findings: _____

Chapter 13 - Postural Analysis

Look in the mirror. Check the height of your ears, shoulders, fingertips, and hips.

Use a ruler to draw a line across the figure below, showing which areas of your body are level and which are not.

This will illustrate any abnormalities in your posture.

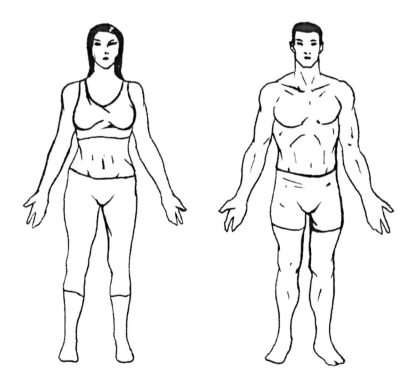

Chapter 14 - Flat Feet

After wetting the bottom of your feet and stepping on a smooth, flat surface, observe the imprints of your feet and record your findings here. If you can see your entire foot, you have flat feet. If your imprint does not show the middle of your foot, you do not suffer from flat feet.

Right Foot:

_____

_____

Left Foot:

_____

_____

Chapter 15 – Proper Breathing

Follow the instructions in Chapter 15 to determine if you are a chest breather or a stomach breather. Fill in the date and place a check mark next to the method used (standing or lying down) and your findings.

Date				
Standing				
Lying Down				
Chest Breather				
Stomach Breather				

Bibliography

Chapter 1

(1) Null, G, PhD, Dean, C, MD, ND, Feldman, M, MD, Rasio, D, MD, Smith, D, PhD. "2004" Death by Medicine. Retrieved May 13, 2012 from Life Extension magazine. www.lef.org/magazine/mag2004/mar2004_awsi_death_01.htm

(2) McKenzie, J. "Conflict of Interest? Medical journal changes policy of finding independent contractors [transcript]. ABC News. June 12, 2002.

(3) Campbell, EG, Weissman JS, Clarridge B, Yucel, R, Causino, N, Blumenthal, D. "Characteristics of Medical School faculty members serving on institutional review boards: results of a national survey". Acad. Med. 2003. Aug; 78(8): 831-6.

Chapter 2

(1) U.S. National Library of Medicine. "2012" High blood pressure. Retrieved May, 14 2012 from Medline Plus www.nlm.nih.gov/medlineplus/highbloodpressure.html

(2) Lancet 2007: 370: 539: Hypertension: uncontrolled and conquering the world. [editorial]

(3) American Heart Association. "2012" High blood pressure. Retrieved May 14, 2012 from American Heart Association www.heart.org/HEARTORG/conditions/HighBloodPressure...re_UCM_301785_Article.jsp

(4) National Heart, Lung, and Blood Institute. "2003" Seventh Report of the Joint National Committee on Prevention, Detection, Evaluation, and Treatment of High Blood Pressure, Retrieved May 14, 2012 from JNC 7 Express http://www.nhlbi.nih.gov/guidelines/hypertension/jhcintro.htm

(5) Rosch, P. "2009" Why has the treatment of hypertension become such a deplorable fiasco? Retrieved May 14, 2012 from The American Institute of Stress www.stress.org/interview-Stress_Hypertension.htm

(6) Heid, M. "2012" The simple test that could save your life. Retrieved May 14, 2012 from Prevention www.prevention.com/health/health-concerns/importance-blood-pressure-testing-both-arms

Chapter 4

(1) Stoppler, M, MD. "2012" Food allergy. Retrieved May 14, 2012 from MedicineNet.com
www.medicinenet.com/food_allergy/article.htm

(2) Coca, A, MD. "1956" The pulse test [online copy]. Retrieved May 14, 2012 from The Soil and Health Library.
www.soilandhealth.org/02/020kyglibcat/020108.coca.pdf

(3) Coca, A, MD. "1956" The pulse test [online copy]. Retrieved May 14, 2012 from The Soil and Health Library.
www.soilandhealth.org/02/020kyglibcat/020108.coca.pdf

Chapter 5

(1) Morgan, S. "2011" Adrenal glands and kidney. Retrieved May 15, 2012 from Livestrong.com www.livesrong.com/article/139350-adrenal-glands-kidneys/

(2) Bartter, FC, Fourman P. "The different effects of aldosterone-like steroids and
hydrocortisone-like steroids on urinary excretion of potassium and acid". Metabolism. 11:6, 1962 [PubMed]

Chapter 6

(1) Bowthorpe, J, M.Ed. "Stop the Thyroid Madness". 2nd Ed. 2011. Ch. 5.

Chapter 7

(1) Mincin, K, Clin. Nut. "2006" Calcium quick test. Retrieved May 15, 2012 from Nutrition Testing.com www.nutrition-testing.com/nutritionresource/testing1.htm

Chapter 8

(1) Sklovsky, R. Pharm. D, ND, PC. "2003" Low thyroid: the unsuspected illness. Retrieved May 15, 2012 from Dr. Bob ND.com
www.drbobnd.com/low_thyroid.htm

Chapter 9

(1) Alternative Medicine Angel. "2000" How to self test for iodine deficiency. Retrieved on May 15, 2012 from Altmedangel.com
http://altmedangel.com/iodine.htm

(2) Goodson, D. "2005" What are the symptoms of hypothyroidism. Retrieved May 15, 2012 from A 2 Z of Health, Beauty, and Fitness
Health.learninginfo.org/hypothyroidism.htm
Health.learninginfo.org/hypothyroidism.htm

Chapter 10

(1)   Cousins, RI. Zinc. In: Present Knowledge in Nutrition. Ed. Zeigler EE, Filer LJ. Washington DC. ILSI Press 1996.

(2)   Sandstead, MW. (2006). "Zinc requirements and the risks and benefits of zinc supplementation". *J Trace Elem Med Biol* **20** (1): 3–18.

(3)   Eby, G. "2011" Warning! Zinc deficiency—as cause of modern illnesses. Retrieved May 16, 2012 from George Eby Research Institute http://george-eby-research.com/html/warning.html

(4)   "Gestational zinc deprivation in mice: persistence of immunodeficiency for three generations". Science. 1982, Vol. 218. 469-471.

(5)   Office of Dietary Supplement. "2011" Dietary supplement fact sheet: zinc". Retrieved May 15, 2012 from National Institute of Health ods.od.nih.gov/factsheets/zinc-HealthProfessional/

Chapter 11

(1)   Simmer K, Thompson RP. Zinc in the fetus and newborn. Acta Paediatr Scand Suppl 1985;319:158-63. [PubMed abstract]

(2)   Rink L, Gabriel P. Zinc and the immune system. Proc Nutr Soc 2000;59:541-52. [PubMed abstract]

(3)   Shankar AH, Prasad AS. Zinc and immune function: the biological basis of altered resistance to infection. Am J Clin Nutr 1998;68:447S-63S. [PubMed abstract]

(4)   Hulisz D. Efficacy of zinc against common cold viruses: an overview. J Am Pharm Assoc (2003) 2004;44:594-603. [PubMed abstract]

Chapter 12

(1)   Intestinal Dysbiosis. "2011" Intestinal dysbiosis: my story. Retrieved May 16, 2012 from Intestinal Dysbiosis.com http://intestinaldysbiosis.com/dysbiosis/dysbacteriosis-symptoms-treatment

(2)   Lipschultz-Robinson, S. "1996" Candida: conquering yeast infections – the non-drug solution. Retrieved on May 16, 2012 from Shirley's Wellness Café http://www.shirleys-wellness-cafe.com/candida.htm

Chapter 14

    (1)   Dr Foot. "1994" Flat feet. Retrieved May 17, 2012 from Dr Foot.co.uk http://www.drfoot.co.uk.htm

Chapter 15

    (1)   "Pulmonary Function is a Long Term Predictor of Mortality in General Population: 29 year follow up of the Buffalo Health Study". [Pubmed]

    (2)   Stop Anxiety Attack Symptoms. "2012" Breathing – the proper technique. Retrieved May 18, 2012 from Stop Anxiety Attack Symptoms.com http://www.stop-anxiety-attack-symptoms.com/breathing.html

    (3)   Rakhimov, A. "2011" Chest (thoracic) breathing: effects, tests, and solutions. Retrieved from Normal Breathing.com http://www.normalbreathing.com/index-chest-breathing.php

    (4)   Peters, D. "2012" Upper chest breathing. Retrieved May 19, 2012 from Murphy's Law Neuromuscular Therapy http://www.murphyslawmassagetherapy.com/upper-chest-breathing

    (5)   Krucoff, C. "Better living through belly breathing". The Seattle Times. May 10, 2000. Section C3

Picture Credits:

The publisher would like to thank the following for their kind permission to reproduce their photographs:

Wikimedia Commons for public Domain Images used in the Header and Footer and on the Cover of this book.

Chapter 2
- (1) Taking Blood Pressure from phil.cdc.gov/phil/quicksearch.asp
- (2) Wrist Cuff from Wikipedia.org File: Blutdruck.jpg

Chapter 3
- (1) Fingertip Pulse Oximeter from Wikipedia.org File: FingertipPulseOximeter_MD3001C1NoLogo.jug

Chapter 4
- (1) How to Take Pulse from Wikipedia.org File: Pulse_evaluation.jpg
- (2) Wrist Blood Pressure Cuff from Wikipedia.org File: Blutdruck.jpg
- (3) Heart Rate Wrist Band from Wikipedia.org File: MF-180.jpg

Chapter 5
- (1) Endocrine System from Wikipedia.org File: IlluendocrinesystemNew.png
- (2) Adrenal Glands and Kidneys from Wikipedia.org File: Illu adrenal gland.jpg

Chapter 6
- (1) Eye With Pupil Constricted from ww.catalog.niddk.nih.gov/ImageLibrary/
- (2) Eye With Pupil Dilated from ww.catalog.niddk.nih.gov/ImageLibrary/

Chapter 9
- (1) Woman With Small Goiter from Wikipedia.org File: Struma001.jpg
- (2) Woman With Large Goiter from Wikipedia.org File: Konemed Stor Struma.jpg

Chapter 10
- (1) Picture 1 White Spot on Fingernail from Wikipedia.org File: Leukonychia.jpg
- (2) Picture 2 White Spot on Fingernail from Wikipedia.org File: Leukonychia2.jpg

Chapter 13
- (1) Side View of Spine from images.niams.nih.gov/ImagesFiles/00001_L.jpg

(2) Scoliosis from Wikipedia.org File: Scoliosis cobb.gif

(3) Images on pages 146 - 148 created by Alexander Phoenix (alexanderphoenix.com)

(4) Human Skeleton Front from Wikipedia.org File: Humanskeletonfronten.svg

(5) Human Skeleton Back from Wikipedia.org File: Humanskeletonbacken.svg

Chapter 14

(1) Bones of Feet from Wikipedia.org File: Gray291.jpg

(2) Foot with Normal Arch from Wikipedial.org File: Male Right Foot 1.jpg

(3) Flat Foot from Wikipedia.org File: Flatfoot.jpg

Appendix B

(1) Images on page 210 created by Alexander Phoenix (alexanderphoenix.com)

About the Author

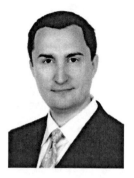

Dr. Vladimir Gordin is a man who needs no introduction. He has been a leading practitioner of Chiropractic and of the healing arts for over a decade. Using methods that show his innate understanding of the human organism, Dr. Gordin has changed the lives of thousands of patients. Dr. Gordin also lectures regularly on health related issues, and has his own highly popular radio show listened to in over 20 countries on five continents.

Dr. Gordin's qualifications include his Doctorate in Chiropractic from the prestigious National University of Health Sciences, his degrees in Biology and Physics and Human Biology, and post-graduate studies that have qualified him to be Board Eligible Diplomate in Chiropractic Orthopedics and Applied Kinesiology, as well as Board Candidate Diplomate in Clinical Nutrition. He also holds certifications that grant him mastery over a large variety of treatment protocols. His qualifications and considerable experience allow Dr. Gordin to use a vast array of highly effective methods and techniques.

*The **core** of Dr. Gordin's **philosophy** is treating the root cause of a patient's problems. His **goal** is to help his patients towards lasting and permanent health, guiding them towards a gentle, yet rapid, recovery.*

This series of books by Dr. Gordin is an expression of this philosophy and goal...

Dr. Gordin resides with his beautiful wife and three children in Chicago, IL.

CPSIA information can be obtained at www.ICGtesting.com
Printed in the USA
LVOW10s2148131113

361176LV00034B/2497/P